THE RENEWAL OF GENEROSITY

Arthur W. Frank

THE RENEWAL OF
Generosity

ILLNESS, MEDICINE, AND HOW TO LIVE

THE
UNIVERSITY
OF CHICAGO
PRESS

☒

Chicago and London

The University of Chicago Press, Chicago 60637
The University of Chicago Press, Ltd., London
© 2004 by The University of Chicago
All rights reserved. Published 2004
Paperback edition 2005
Printed in the United States of America

19 18 17 16 15 14 13 12 11 10 09   3 4 5 6 7 8

ISBN-13: 978-0-226-26015-0 (cloth)
ISBN-13: 978-0-226-26017-4 (paper)
ISBN-10: 0-226-26015-1 (cloth)
ISBN-10: 0-226-26017-8 (paper)

Library of Congress Cataloging-in-Publication Data

Frank, Arthur W.
The renewal of generosity: illness, medicine, and how to live /
Arthur W. Frank.
    p. ; cm.
Includes bibliographical references and index.
ISBN 0-226-26015-1 (hardcover : alk. paper)
1. Physician and patient.   2. Generosity.
[DNLM: 1. Physician-Patient Relations.   2. Empathy.   3. Ethics, Medical.
W 62 F828r 2004]   I. Title.
R727.3 .F66 2004
610.69'6—dc21   2003011971

In *The Possessed,* Shatov tells Stavrogin:
"[W]e are two *beings,* and have come
together *in infinity* . . . for the *last time in the
world.* Drop your tone, and speak like a
human being! Speak, if only for once in
your life, with the voice of a man."

All decisive encounters of man with man,
consciousness with consciousness, always
take place in Dostoevsky's novels
"in infinity" and "for the last time"
(in the ultimate moments of crisis).
MIKHAIL BAKHTIN,
Problems in Dostoevsky's Poetics

What then does one seek?
Not a hidden power,
but a source of kinship for mature persons.
And also the assurance that it is
not totally absurd to have suffered.
EMMANUEL LEVINAS,
Is It Righteous to Be?

None of us is forbidden to pursue
our own good.
MARCUS AURELIUS, *Meditations*

CONTENTS

INTRODUCTION
A Hospitable Welcome
1

ONE
Lost in the Tunnel
12

TWO
The Dialogical Stoic
30

THREE
The Generosity of the Ill
55

FOUR
Physicians' Generosity
78

FIVE
"So that I can carry on"
106

SIX
Unfinalized Generosity
123

Acknowledgments
145

Notes   *Index*
147   163

A Hospitable Welcome

A PHYSICIAN once asked me if I had ever expressed "unqualified gratitude" to the doctors who treated me when I had cancer. I hadn't. The other side of the question is how often I felt that I was being cared for with unqualified generosity. Not often enough. I regret that, for us all.

> *You've wandered all over and finally realized that you never found what you were after: how to live.*
> MARCUS AURELIUS
>
> ❀

What went wrong, on both sides? How can there be a renewal of generosity and a reciprocal increase in gratitude? How could a renewal of generosity among the ill and those who care for them resonate through the human community? We humans seem to be most generous when we feel grateful and desire to pass on some measure of what we have been given. Medical care can play a privileged role in this cycle of generosity, gratitude, and more generosity. Medical generosity sets a standard for the rest of society, because illness is a universal form of suffering.

This book is about what I consider *fundamental* medicine: face-to-face encounters between people who are suffering bodily ills and other people who need both the skills to relieve this suffering and the grace to welcome those who suffer. Medical generosity lies in that latter quality—the grace to welcome those who suffer. My conviction is that at the start of the twenty-first century, the foremost task of responding to illness and disability is not devising new treatments, though I'm grateful this work will proceed. Our challenge is to increase the generosity with which we offer the medical skill that has been attained. Pharmaceuticals and surgeries, diagnostic techniques and institutional provision of services are crucial tools of medical work, but in this book I leave these in the background. Before and after these tools, medicine

1

is people in a room together, acting toward each other with varying degrees of generosity.

Before and after fundamental medicine offers diagnoses, drugs, and surgery to those who suffer, it should offer consolation. Consolation is a gift. Consolation comforts when loss occurs or is inevitable. This comfort may be one person's promise not to abandon another. Consolation may render loss more bearable by inviting some shift in belief about the point of living a life that includes suffering. Thus consolation implies a period of transition: a preparation for a time when the present suffering will have turned. Consolation promises that turning.

To offer consolation is an act of generosity.

Generosity begins in *welcome:* a hospitality that offers whatever the host has that would meet the need of the guest. The welcome of opening the doors of one's home signifies the opening the self to others, including guests who may disrupt and demand. To guests who suffer, the host's welcome is an initial promise of consolation. If the cosmic creation of life is the founding act of generosity, the human gift of consolation has at least one analogous quality: no reciprocity is required, for indeed none may be possible.

When the giving of consolation is taken to be the paradigm of generosity, our imagination of what might be a generous relationship moves beyond material gifts and the economy of exchange that material gifts instigate. Generosity transcends any expectation for what the gift may bring back in reciprocity. Generosity implies the host's trust in the renewable capacity to give; the generous person feels no need to measure what is given against what is received. Generosity does not plan for the giver's own future. It responds to the guest's need.

Yet because what is offered can never meet the guest's need completely, the welcome that generosity offers contains a plea for forgiveness. The biblical story of Job's three friends, who arrive to console him and stay to accuse him, reminds us that consolation will always go wrong to some degree, and generosity always falls short.

Generosity accepts our ultimate human failure to be generous. What counts is continuing to reopen the door of hospitality, welcoming the guest who needs consolation.[1]

⌘

THE traditional ideal of medicine is to offer more than treatment. The hospitality that exceeds treatment welcomes the sick person without qualification. Medical hospitality invites the ill to feel less stigmatized and isolated. According to this ancient ideal, those who make medicine their work are to find their consolation in being the kind of people who offer such hospitality.

A shadowy figure who gives a name to the ideal of medical generosity is described by Jerome, writing in 399 about one of his disciples. He describes a woman called Fabiola—a name I value for its suggestion of some extrahuman quality. Fabiola seems not quite of this world.

She was the first person to found a hospital into which she might gather sufferers out of the streets and where she may nurse the unfortunate victims of sickness and want. Need I speak of noses slit, eyes put out, feet half burned, hands covered with sores? Or of limbs dropsical and atrophied? Or of diseased flesh alive with worms? Often did she carry on her shoulders persons infected with jaundice or filth. Often too did she wash away the matter discharged from the wounds which others, even though men, could not bear to look at. She gave food to her patients with her own hand, and moistened the scarce breathing lips of the dying with sips of liquid.[2]

Fabiola's example of saintly generosity was compromised long before modern medicine. Medical historian Guenter Risse notes that medieval Benedictine monastic hostels received the poor and the wealthy in different quarters, despite the ideal of hospitality established by chapter 36 of The Rule of St. Benedict: "before all things and above all things special care must be taken of the sick or infirm so that they may be served as if they were Christ in person" (96). The conflict between hospitality and practicality is as old as organized medicine. Practical lack of resources is immediately complicated by possibilities of financial gain. As early as 1130, monks were prohibited from practicing medicine, because it might interfere with their spiritual vocation. "By 1219," Risse writes, "canon law again prohibited religious persons from practicing medicine because of the monetary gain it brought" (153). By the fourteenth century, Fabiola's children encountered managed care: "Hospitals were now forced to ration their caregiving through better screening of applicants. . . . Throughout Europe, hospital authorities now worried about admitting too many poor people with chronic conditions who would occupy most beds for long periods of time—a costly proposition" (154). Thus "Some overseers of a hospital's revenues [came to view] their tasks as an ordinary business instead of a charitable, spiritually rewarding enterprise" (155).

To the perennial conflict between Fabiola's spirit of hospitality and the tendency of organized medicine to become a business, this book seeks to offer consolation. I present stories of how ill people and clinicians renew generosity in medicine. My work is to show how these stories ought to count for more people, more of the time. Thus I bring stories together to reinforce each by its complementarity with others. In turn, these stories are complemented by fragments of mostly philosophical theory that connect specific problems of particular people with generalized problems of humanity. Medicine is, I believe, a privileged site at which to reflect on such problems.

Medical care both sets and reflects standards for caring relationships between individuals in a society. By this overused word *care*, I mean an occasion when people discover what each can be in relationship with the other. Too many people in medical settings, patients and staff both, are isolated from one another even as they work, suffer, and hope in the most intimate synchrony. One eloquent testimony to this loneliness-in-proximity is offered by physician Abraham Verghese at the end of his meditation on the life of a younger physician friend who killed himself through his drug addiction. Verghese argues, perhaps even pleads, that rate of substance abuse among doctors is indicative of what medicine does to its practitioners:

Despite all our grand societies, memberships, fellowships, specialty colleges, each with its annual dues and certificates and ceremonials, we are horribly alone. The doctor's world is one where our own feelings—particularly those of pain and hurt—are not easily expressed, even though *patients* are encouraged to express them. We trust our colleagues, we show propriety and reciprocity, we have the scientific knowledge, we learn empathy, but we rarely expose our own emotions.[3]

What Verghese says about doctors I can repeat, from years of personal experience, about patients. Despite all the support groups, the ribbons and teddy bears, the urban festivals of runs and walks for different cures, and (less frequent) memorials, people go through illness feeling alone too much of the time.[4] Verghese writes that patients are encouraged to express their feelings, and a variety of venues for such expressions are available. But in both clinics and peer support groups—both face to face and on the Internet—these expressions are constrained by norms encouraging, and sometimes requiring, what counts as hope, humor, and a "positive attitude." Expressions of pain, bafflement, and despair are rarely welcome; at best they produce group confusion, at worst they are ostracized. Thus patients, like doctors, spend so much time presenting the emotions required by different situations that they lose their sense of what they do feel. Patients, like medical staff, feel a lack of generosity.

I recall a woman who had a rare cancer, which was cured after extensive treatment. She and her partner described their experience as surviving the cancer but barely surviving the treatment center. Saying and repeating that description brought them some consolation, and they needed to be consoled for the treatment center's lack of hospitality. But this consolation was not generous; it was divisive, not healing. Their experience, expressed by many ill people, is complemented by conversations I have had with various physicians, generally at night, in a car, when my host was driving me back to my hotel after a long day's conference. During that day I'd gotten to know this person enough to admire him (these have always been men, but that says less about gender divisions in medicine than it says about me as an object of people's confessional impulses). I'd come to think of this physician as someone I would like to have taking care of me and my family, because I sensed that he truly does care for his patients, in excess of whatever treatment he offers them. Then he said, and it startled me, that he's thinking seriously of quitting medicine, maybe for an extended sabbatical, maybe permanently.

These physicians have trouble articulating their reasons for quitting: it's not the money, certainly not the patients, and not even any specific conditions of work. The whole medical scene has become antithetical to what the physician realizes he needs to be the person he wants to be. These physicians know they are doing good, important work that serves others, but they feel that something crucial to who they are is being destroyed in the process. I want to help these doctors imagine how they could go on practicing medicine *and* be the people they want to be. This book extends that imagining, just as I hope it offers consolation to patients who have barely survived their treatments. These dual consolations—to patients and medical professionals—can be effective only in tandem. Neither can be consoled unless the other is.

Fabiola had more ability to welcome than she had skills or resources to cure, but Jerome depicts her as unfailingly generous in offering consolation. Her generosity was her willingness to clean wounds that others could not bear to look at. She touched those whom others feared to touch. Fabiola's touch was both literal and metaphoric, exemplifying how care is enacted in gestures that can console far beyond what they accomplish as practical components of treatment. For touch to console and thus to heal, it must be more than efficient. Touch must be generous, seeking contact with a person as much as it seeks to effect some task. Generosity is the resonance of touch, endowing the act with a capacity to give beyond its practical significance. There is no reason why the skilled touch cannot also be generous. On the contrary, true skill has to include generosity.

The sick and injured whom Fabiola rescued from the streets of Rome in late antiquity certainly would have had their medical needs better served in a contemporary emergency room, but we cannot imagine them being *welcomed* as she welcomed them. To force a choice between either the skills of the contemporary hospital or Fabiola's generosity is to freeze each in what it lacks and force choosing between what we would rather do without. This book refuses that choice. It offers an alternative: to learn from the ill people and medical professionals whose stories show how to be generous.

⁜

YOU'VE *wandered all over and finally realized that you never found what you were after: how to live.* So wrote the Stoic philosopher and Roman emperor Marcus Aurelius.[5] In its professional persona, medicine has wandered as far inside the human body as molecular biology can penetrate. It wanders through treatment and research complexes the size of cities. But the further medicine wanders and the more expansive its concerns become, the more it poses Marcus's question of what we—both those who practice medicine and those whose lives are constantly measured, assessed, and documented by medical standards—are after: *how to live?*

If Marcus could not find how to live, of course I haven't either. But I have collected stories about people finding a good deal of what they are after, and learning to recognize what gets in the way of what they seek. I do not analyze these stories. I advocate trying to think *with* them, a process closer to letting the stories analyze us. Stories analyze us by allowing us to notice what attracts us to them, and what we resist about them. They show us what we want, and ask us what we need. We begin to think *with* stories when situations in our lives recall these accounts so often that they settle into our awareness and become habits of thought, tacitly guiding our actions.

Stories stand better together, each increasing the resonance of others like it. The literary scholar Northrop Frye defined *resonance* as how "a particular statement in a particular context acquires a universal significance."[6] This "universal significance" of stories is not some truth for all times and places. It's their ability to pose questions and offer examples that inform lives lived far from the story's particular time and place. The examples that stories offer—their heroes—do not tell readers what to do; rather they are examples of struggling to figure out what has to be done and gathering the resolve to go about doing it. The stories in this book do not prescribe: "*this* is generosity." Storytellers work to discover what it means to be generous where they are, facing what they face. Their struggles, including their uncertainty, are their resonance. We read them from where we are, in our uncertainty, facing what we face.

Most of all, the stories exemplify the seriousness of people who seek what they are after: how to live. The stories, unlike case studies in clinical ethics journals, are not models of correct responses to dilemmas, told so that others can act that way in similar situations. They teach us how to be serious about how we act wherever we find ourselves. If they are models of anything, the stories model moral sensitivity to what makes each situation unique and each decision difficult. These stories contain no hidden or coded meanings that require analysis; they speak clearly for themselves. But how to hear the stories—neither to decode them nor to admire them but to make them part of our own practices of generosity—does require reflection.

I invite readers to hear the philosophical fragments that complement the stories as if they were spoken by what contemporary family therapy calls a reflecting team. A therapeutic reflecting team consists of the therapist's supervisors and colleagues who sit behind a one-way mirror and watch the therapy session. Sometimes they telephone the therapist who sits with the family on the other side of the mirror, suggesting possible questions to ask. Sometimes they come into the therapy room, and the family and therapist take a turn behind the mirror to watch the reflecting team talk about what they see happening.

Reflecting teams do not offer analyses or judgments, diagnostic or otherwise. As their name implies, they reflect. Practices of reflection vary, but reflecting teams offer themselves as a kind of mirror, in which family and therapist can see their lives reflected in a new language and new images.[7] A good reflecting team expands people's sense of who they are and who they could be. It is in this spirit that I offer philosophical fragments to expand the significance of the stories I tell, and how they could change lives.

Reflecting teams do observe certain conventions. They do not debate their differences among themselves; the focus must remain on the family's story as it is enacted before them. Debate among members of the reflecting team can take place later. Deferring debate—staying focused on the lived story—will clarify the theoretical stakes. Another practice of reflecting teams is to limit the number of voices when they take their place in front of the mirror and offer their reflections, lest too many voices blur the impact of the reflections. My literary and philosophical reflecting team follows both practices. I try to quote those whose help I need only so far as I need them to reflect on some story, I try not to address theories to each other or engage in critique of their ideas, and I limit the number of voices in order to focus on the stories.

I call my reflecting team the Dialogical Stoic, an odd usage that will be explained in chapter 2. The Dialogical Stoic is emphatically not an ism. The reflections are neither a system of thought nor a theoretical framework—an unfortunate phrase that suggests the stories need containing. To resist such imputations, I present the Dialogical Stoic as a persona, though that usage has its own problems. The Dialogical Stoic is not a unified persona but a collection of voices that remain distinct. A clinical reflecting team is, literally, a crowded room full of voices that speak from different perspectives but share commitments about how human life works and what's good for humans. The voices that fill the Dialectical Stoic provide resonant reflections on what is good in stories about illness, medicine, and care.

The Dialogical Stoic reflects on how to *live with* illness, disability, and death. Medicine from Fabiola to the present has sought to *resist* the fate of our bodies' vulnerability. If we have not yet reached the limit of that project, we may have reached a threshold where the enterprise turns against itself. The bodily vulnerability that medicine resists with honorable dedication is part of what humans *are;* not a

contingent and undesired side effect of being human—a wart to be removed—but part of what it is to be human, warts and all. Thus medicine, in its dedication to the human goal of reducing suffering, always
risks rejecting a fundamental aspect of our humanity. Medicine, not in
its mistakes but in its noblest intentions, can inadvertently increase
suffering. We whose lives are dependent on medicine and whose
thinking is thoroughly imbued with medical values risk failing to explore the significance of an idea utterly heretical to medicine: that as a
species, and as individuals, we may need to be ill.

We fail to console ourselves with the recognition that illness may
be necessary to realize all we can become as humans. Humanity needs
to cure illness when it can. But that need can blind us to an equally important goal: how do we accommodate our lives to what we can never
cure, ultimately death? Accommodating illness has never been easy,
either as an attitude toward life or as a practical problem. Even for the
medieval Benedictines, as assured of their faith as we (perhaps nostal-
gically) would like to imagine them, how hospitality was actually offered—what it meant in practice to receive each guest as if she or he
were Christ in person—nonetheless required decisions about how to
arrange the rooms and who could stay in which bed for how long. For
those most dedicated to the good, what constitutes the good is never
given in advance. Stories can guide us in thinking seriously about what
we seek, and what values we seek to preserve in our seeking.

The resonance of stories is what they give beyond what they
ostensibly tell. Stories of the generosity of ill people, doctors, and
nurses can show what is possible for any of us at any time. That is their
consolation.

※

CHAPTER 1 begins with a story that shows how subtle the withholding
of generosity in medicine can be, even when treatment seems exemplary. Some shorter stories then depict generosity being renewed.
Chapter 2 introduces the Dialogical Stoic: who is on my reflecting
team, and why each has something important to say about illness and
care. This delayed introduction of the Dialogical Stoic is another gesture marking that the book is not about those on the reflecting team;
the philosophers are there to reflect on the stories and give them more
resonance. Chapter 3 tells stories of how ill people and their families
turn illness into an occasion for generosity. Chapter 4 tells comple-

mentary stories about physicians: how they seek to change themselves, and medicine, by renewing generosity. Chapter 5 narrows the focus to a single interview excerpt in which a palliative care nurse describes the care of one patient. The chaotic uncertainty of generosity in practice can be felt in this narrative, which has none of the retrospective closure of the stories told in chapter 4. Chapter 6 poses dilemmas of practicing generosity within institutions that impose impersonal demands, and the Dialogical Stoic offers final reflections.

A central issue throughout this book is how the ill and disabled are represented in language, and three issues of my own language use deserve mention. The first issue involves my unsuccessful attempt to root out all usage of the substantive noun *medicine* as the subject of some verb ("medicine causes . . . "). Medicine today comprises an unthinkably broad array of knowledge and skills, professions, coalitions, and interest groups, fears and promises, fantasies and soon-to-be-realities, concrete and virtual institutions, folklores and sciences. Parts of this array enter people's awareness, and other parts affect them outside their awareness. Yet as diffuse as medicine is, the substantive noun *medicine*—with its pernicious illusion that unitary enterprise exists—proves unavoidable. When I refer to medicine, I mean contextual factors that make a difference when two human persons meet and act toward each other. Context matters, but it's not fate. The stories I tell are about people trying to do something with the contexts in which they find themselves. They are stories about how to use medicine, and how to be used by it as little as possible.

The second issue involves pronouns. I try to write in a voice of direct address—speaking to *you* rather than writing of *them*, and of *us* rather than *one*. This book is not about other people: sooner or later we all will be ill or disabled, and we all are called to offer care, whether as professionals, volunteers, friends, or family members. The renewal of generosity requires envisioning this vast enterprise of care for suffering as one in which we all participate together, each doing his or her part that would be impossible without others doing their parts. *We* is a constant reminder of our engagement and our interdependence.

A third language problem is the proliferation of terms designating patients (also known as ill and disabled people; sometimes designated as consumers) and medical workers (known by professional designations; generically designated as providers). My preferred terms are *guests* (those needing care) and *hosts* (those temporarily in a position to offer care, including people whose main qualification is their own illness or disability). The renewal of generosity will be hastened if participants in medical relationships think of themselves not (at least not only) as patients and professionals, much less as consumers and providers, but as guests and hosts. Those terms will not always fit in the chapters that follow, but I hope to use them often enough to recall and expand their significance.

CHAPTER ONE

Lost in the Tunnel

A DOCTOR recalls a haunting incident from his early professional
life in his story "The Tunnel." The tunnel is a metaphor of both illness and
medical relationships. In the course of
any serious illness, patients and doctors
go through their own tunnel together.
The story poses the problem of who they
will be for each other as they take this
shared journey. In this story the physician and patient are not host and guest,
nor does the story's author seem to imagine such a relationship. Instead, "The
Tunnel" depicts the sort of medical practice that those who tell the stories in later
chapters are trying to change.

"The Tunnel" appears in a little book
with a provocative title, *When a Doctor
Hates a Patient and Other Chapters in a
Young Physician's Life,* coauthored by the late Enid Rhodes Peschel,
who was codirector of the medical humanities program at Yale Medical School, and Richard Peschel, a radiologist. Each chapter begins with
a story told in the first person by Richard Peschel, describing some
incident in his medical residency and early career. Enid Peschel then
discusses various literary texts that expand the issues in Richard's
story. The book seems intended primarily for teaching medical students; because the story is presented as a teaching vehicle, I feel comfortable scrutinizing it. I'd offer Richard Peschel the benefit of the
doubt that he is presenting the example of his younger self so student
physicians can consider better ways of acting in similar situations.

> *The very being of
> man . . . is* deepest
> communion. To be
> *means to* communicate.
> *Absolute death (non-
> being) is the state of
> being unheard,
> unrecognized,
> unremembered. To be
> means to be for another,
> and through the other,
> for oneself. A person has
> no internal sovereignty,
> he is wholly and always
> on the boundary;
> looking inside of himself,
> he looks* into the eyes of
> another *or with the eyes
> of another.*
> MIKHAIL BAKHTIN
>
> ⌘

The story begins as many medical tales do. It's 2:00 A.M. and young Peschel is just going to sleep in the on-call room. He is called to the emergency room to admit Mr. B, a patient who has a history of heart attacks and may be having another one now. Peschel must transport Mr. B from the emergency room to the Coronary Care Unit, which is in another building of the same hospital. The emergency room and morgue are in an older building that is joined to the newer facility by a tunnel. Here's part of Peschel's evocation of how surreal the connecting tunnel is:

The tunnel is like no other. It is long and narrow (approximately one and one-half city blocks from end to end and two stretchers wide). Its gray cement floor looks worn, as though scarred with the weight of all the feet and wheels that have hurried over its sunless surface. . . . It is difficult to breathe even if you are healthy and not in distress like the patient on the stretcher. The only sound you hear is the droning of the ventilation fan. You wonder if it is really working, the air is so stale. . . . Fluorescent tubes fling down light from above and make you squint. Except for one curve, the tunnel is straight. If you stare directly ahead, you think you are caught in an almost endless tube.[1]

Peschel first takes the time to do just what he should: reassure Mr. B and offer some pain relief. He then begins to accompany Mr. B and a considerable amount of monitoring gear through the tunnel.

Coming toward them from the far end of the tunnel is what Peschel first perceives as "an apparition . . . a caravan of several black-clad shapes advancing slowly" (12). Mr. B sees only the ceiling. As these shapes get closer, Peschel realizes they are men transporting a body from the main hospital to the morgue, but the scene is wrong: these are not hospital workers, nor are they using the hospital-issue blue box for transporting the body.

I realize that the procession is composed of a number of bearded fellows garbed in black hats and black outfits—everything about them seems black. . . . The caravan['s] mournful and foreboding mien makes it look like a cortege from hell. It is terrifying to me, and I am perfectly sound. (12–13)

Peschel hopes Mr. B will not see the procession, but at the crucial moment when the two gurneys pass, almost touching each other in the narrow tunnel, Mr. B turns his head and faces the corpse. "No one says a word," Peschel writes. "I keep looking at Mr. B. He is still as stone. At last he looks up at me. And I know, from nothing but the expression on his face, that he believes he has just seen an image of himself. We do not talk. We barely breathe" (12–13).

They make it to the Coronary Care Unit, Mr. B survives what was in fact another heart attack, and Peschel continues as one of his physicians. One day, as Mr. B is getting ready for discharge, he asks Peschel if what he saw was a dead body. Peschel's exact choice of words seems crucial here: "I cannot escape answering. 'Yes, it was,' I respond. That is all that happened. We did not talk more about it, then or ever" (13–14).

Weeks later, Peschel learns that what they saw was a group of Orthodox Jews who had received permission to accompany a distinguished rabbi to the morgue as part of their ritual vigil over his body. The ritual includes draping the body in a sheet instead of placing it inside one of the blue boxes used by the hospital. The rest of the chapter rehearses depictions of death in literature, from Montaigne to Tolstoy to Solzhenitsyn. No reflection is offered on the care that the young Richard Peschel offered his patient. Instead, "the memory of the cortege and [his] patient's face continues to haunt" Peschel whenever he walks through the tunnel (14). He does not wonder what might haunt Mr. B, and what he might have done to relieve Mr. B's confusion, both in the tunnel and later.

MEDICAL DEMORALIZATION

The tunnel is an evocative metaphor of the experience of being ill. Stories of being diagnosed as having a life-threatening or life-altering illness—deep illness that casts its shadow over the person's whole future—often use metaphors of suddenly finding oneself in a tunnel-like space where it's difficult to breathe, the light is blinding and distorting, any possibility of movement seems caught in an inescapable track, and ominously unknown shapes are coming out of the distance. Barbara Rosenblum suggests being in a psychic tunnel as she evokes her receiving a diagnosis of breast cancer. Even a diagnosis that she was prepared to expect throws her into shock:

I shut my eyes and saw absolute black, no lines of red or purple, pure black. My agitation lifted me off the table and I started walking around the examination room in small steps, working off the tension. I thought I might put my fist through the wall.

And then, when I opened my eyes, I couldn't see too well. Or hear too well either. Anna, my good friend who was with me, took the notes, handled the paperwork . . . escorted me through the distorted corridors of the hospital, and finally drove me home.[2]

As Rosenblum tells this story, her physician becomes a disembodied voice; he never enters the tunnel she is in. Rosenblum is lucky to have Anna. Mr. B has Peschel.

The tunnel is an equally evocative metaphor for institutional medicine: the organizational and physical structures within which care is offered. Medicine can seem to be a constricting space that makes it difficult to see things in their proper light and to talk about what these things mean. Hospitals are experienced as what Rosenblum calls "distorted corridors." Medical institutions can be spaces like Peschel's tunnel that seem to embody nightmares.

Arthur Kleinman, in his classic book *The Illness Narratives*, writes that medicine demoralizes: "the contribution of professional orthodoxy to inadvertently heighten the passivity and demoralization of patients and their families is all too common in the treatment of the chronically ill."[3] Not only do the effects of disease demoralize the patient, medical treatment itself demoralizes. This demoralization extends to medical professionals: "we should be critical of a therapeutic method that dehumanizes the doctor along with the patient," Kleinman states (136).

A complementary description of what Kleinman calls demoralization and dehumanization is offered by philosopher Emmanuel Levinas. Speaking of totalitarian regimes, Levinas refers to "the degeneration of generosity,"[4] a phrase that led to the title of this book. Demoralization and the degeneration of generosity each feed the other. Kleinman's demoralized medicine refers to relationships that have ceased to be generous, either to patients or to professionals.

Demoralization means more than low morale. We revisit the perennial conflict between Fabiola's saintly generosity and the Benedictines' need to limit their medical hospitality, before anyone imagined medicine as a business. What began when the Benedictines received the poor and the wealthy in different rooms has become the absence of any moral vision of human obligation. Bioethicist Stephen Lammers describes medicine's demoralization as the inevitable result of economic rationality filling the void of moral purpose:

Instead of thinking about our duties to others, we think of ourselves, and no one is empowered to tell us otherwise. If we have the funds, then we can determine the limits of our medical care; if we do not have the funds, then it is too bad, but we have no say. It is one of the unfortunate side effects of medicine becoming a business that it has lost the moral power it once had in people's lives. There is no sense that nurses and physicians might have anything to teach us about the limits of what might be accomplished through their disciplines.[5]

Lammers's regret that medicine has lost its "moral power" is controversial on two grounds. First is the historical question of how much moral power medicine ever had, as opposed to how other groups used medicine as a means to cloak their agendas in a moral claim of health. The history of medical abuses raised by that question leads to a second objection: is it desirable for medicine to exercise moral power? The counterargument to Lammers is that medicine serves best when it keeps its moral sights low. Nurses and physicians may be most useful, and most humane, when they do their technical work and abstain from moral intervention in their patients' lives.[6]

Lammers's argument for what can be called moral medicine recalls the spirited defense of "moral fiction" by poet, novelist, and essayist John Gardner. Lammers might claim as an ideal for medicine what Gardner claims for art:

True art is *by its nature* moral. We recognize true art by its careful, thoroughly honest search for and analysis of values. It is not didactic because, instead of teaching by authority and force, it explores, open-mindedly, to learn what it should teach. It clarifies, like an experiment in a chemistry lab, and confirms. As a chemist's experiment tests the laws of nature and dramatically reveals the truth or falsity of scientific hypotheses, moral art tests values and rouses trustworthy feelings about the better and the worse in human action.[7]

Clinical practice seems by its nature moral, because how people treat other people necessarily expresses values. Which values are relevant, and how they apply, can be discovered only in practice. Clinical practice can be what Gardner calls a "thoroughly honest search for and analysis of values." The moral clinician does not enter the consultation knowing what values apply and how; that would be "teaching by authority and force." The generous clinician, the host, meets a patient in order to learn and to clarify, in that encounter, what are "trustworthy feelings about the better and worse in human action."

As necessary as Gardner believes moral fiction to be, he recognizes that contemporary nervousness over moral claims reflects bitter historical experience. Moral standards have "frequently been used as a means of oppression, a cover, in some quarters, for political tyranny, self-righteous brutality, hypocrisy, and failed imagination" (46). When monks were enjoined from practicing medicine, not only were they saved from distractions to their spiritual pursuits. Their patients were saved from the potential tyranny of the monks making acceptance of their faith a precondition for receiving their care.

These significant objections show that moral medicine can go wrong; they do not show that medicine can be practiced without moral entanglements. Peschel *is* in the tunnel with Mr. B, and what happens calls for response. How Peschel acts toward Mr. B is a moral problem, not a scientific one. The physician's calling is always both scientific—Peschel must monitor Mr. B's heart—and moral—Peschel also must guide Mr. B through an encounter with death. Lammers's recommendation that medical hosts have something to teach "about the limits of what might be accomplished through their disciplines" points toward a vision of medicine assuming the modest, self-reflecting, experimental morality that Gardner advocates for fiction. A generous response to Mr. B might have ended with a reflection on the limits of medicine.

The question is not whether medicine once had some moral power that it has lost. The pressing contemporary issue is what kind of medical practice could exercise a responsible moral authority that would not be a cover for oppression but would seek continually to learn what it should teach. The examples of generosity assembled in this book offer a middle path between the absence of any moral center that Lammers objects to—the absence that attends demoralization—and, at the other extreme, the potential tyranny of moralism that Gardner recognizes. A generous medicine would necessarily develop the moral sensitivity of hosts and guests as they explore their mutual obligations. To finesse that exploration is to remain lost in the tunnel.

This chapter now returns to the tunnel: first to explore how medicine demoralizes the professional, Peschel; then how it demoralizes the patient, Mr. B; and finally how this demoralization affects the society in which medicine sets a moral standard for how people care for one another. Lest all this writing about demoralization become demoralizing, this chapter concludes with two stories about how medicine can also remoralize. That potential for remoralization is the renewal of generosity.

THE TUNNEL AS MORAL MOMENT

As evocative as Peschel's imagery of the tunnel is, his most haunting words may be his description of how he feels when Mr. B asks him who they passed in the tunnel: "I cannot escape answering." Why, I ask myself in my naïve, nonmedical way, should answering this obvious question—what happened to us back there?—be anything that anyone feels a need to *escape*? As I contemplate this question, a gulf widens between my sense of how any morally and communicatively competent person would respond in such a situation and Peschel's description of how he believed he had to behave as a physician. *Escape* implies more than beliefs about the decorum of who discusses what with whom. Escape is a physical need to get one's body away from some threat. How does Peschel's patient, Mr. B, become such a threat? Peschel answers Mr. B, acknowledging that they passed a dead body, but then he does escape: "We did not talk more about it, then or ever." This concluding statement shows that the choice of the verb, *escape*, was not accidental. Peschel says what he feels.

Mr. B's question creates what physician and philosopher Paul Komesaroff calls a microethical moment. Komesaroff argues, as others have, that an ethics of clinical behavior based on broad principles[8] is "unable to provide an adequate account of day-to-day decision making in medicine," and thus "cannot provide any substantial guidance for medical practice."[9] Komesaroff describes medical practice as "a series of practical tasks" that include, from the physician's side, "the most appropriate way to approach the patient, to talk with him, to allay his fears, and to establish the common ground on which mutual decisions can be taken" (63). These tasks have their complementary responsibilities on the patient's side of the relationship. Thus for both physician and patient, the clinical encounter involves a "continuous flow of ethical decisions," especially over "the degree of openness" that each will adopt toward the other (69). Komesaroff's current research includes analyzing video recordings of physician-patient encounters and attempting to isolate moments of ethical decision making.[10] Mr. B's question is such a moment.

Ethical may not be the best word to describe what happens between

Peschel and Mr. B, since ethics often refers to matters of principle, as in a code of ethics, while *moral* refers to interpersonal, locally contextualized, moment-to-moment actions. But as I wrote this book and considered different authors' uses of *ethical* and *moral*, I found it impossible to sustain a separation between the two words. Let me call Mr. B's question a *moral moment:* an occasion when we must respond to another person, and the nature of that response declares our moral self. Moral moments are frequently ones we would like to "escape," to use Peschel's word, because we sense that how we act will declare who we are. We seek to escape seeing ourselves mirrored in our action. But then the mirror shows us seeking to escape—the moral moment cannot be evaded.

Peschel, as I interpret his story, wants to escape what his response to Mr. B will show about who he is, or about who he has become as a physician. He wants to escape how he felt while he was in the tunnel: uncertain, without resources, alone. Mr. B's question revives those feelings. Peschel's desire for escape reflects his demoralization and perpetuates it. Even in the calm of Mr. B's room, with Mr. B ready for discharge, Peschel does not imagine sharing his feelings with Mr. B. He says as little as possible and retreats into silence. But his silence is a response. The more silent the physician is, the more the relationship between physician and patient becomes a tunnel, and the more constricting that tunnel becomes.

As long as I have considered what Peschel does not want to talk about, the less satisfactory any single explanation seems—can a physician be embarrassed that people die in a hospital? Can he imagine that Mr. B does not realize that people die? Or is it unacceptable for him to allow death to enter into a conversation with a patient? Or, what may be the most troublesome explanation: does Peschel consider that patients are not people whom he can talk *with* about a strange experience they have shared? Can Mr. B, as a patient, only be someone whom Peschel, as a physician, talks *at?* Peschel talks to Mr. B in the emergency room, where he takes time to reassure Mr. B that the situation is under control. But Peschel retains control of this talk; he initiates and directs it. In contrast to this kind of talk, Mr. B's question about what happened in the tunnel is not a patient's request for medical information. The question calls upon the physician to enter into dialogue with someone who at that moment is no longer a patient. Mr. B asks his question as another human being who has had his own experience of the same reality that the physician, his host, experienced. *Dialogue* suggests that the world is coexperienced by two or more people. Each one's perspective is necessarily partial, and each needs to gain a more adequate sense of the world by sharing perspectives.

Peschel and Mr. B have a singular opportunity for dialogue because as the black cortege approaches them, the physician knows the fear that patients live with throughout their stays in hospital. At a moment when two human beings share feelings of uncertainty, lack of resources, and loneliness, dialogue is most possible between them. At such moments, as expressed in this book's first epigraph, it is possible for each to drop his tone and speak with a human voice. But Peschel feels the need to escape. He is too demoralized to seize the moment when dialogue, as a gesture of generosity, is possible and required.

Peschel's avoidance of dialogue evades the principle of human existence stated by this chapter's epigraph. To exist as a human is to communicate with others. Who we can be, any self we can claim, is formed in others' visions of us. The next chapter will introduce Mikhail Bakhtin and his moral ideal of dialogue. For now it suffices to note that while the young physician in the story is doubtless already skilled at presenting his patients in medical rounds and speaking *about* them, he cannot drop that tone and speak *with* Mr. B as one human voice responding to another. In many situations, this lack of engagement in dialogue might pass unnoticed. The tunnel, by its dead air and inescapable light, demands rethinking what is required to live. The only means of life in the tunnel is what Bakhtin calls deepest communion: "to be means to be for another, and through the other."

We can now grasp what makes the medical moment moral. When Peschel cuts off dialogue with Mr. B, he renders both of them "unheard, unrecognized, unremembered," to quote again from this chapter's epigraph. The actual corpse in the tunnel raises the topic of death. The ensuing silence *enacts* death as nonbeing, the opposite of the communion that we can imagine among the men who attend their deceased rabbi: communion they feel with one another and with the body of their spiritual leader.

Peschel's escape from a dialogue in which he could find some communion with Mr. B is also an escape from himself. Medical training has prepared Peschel to believe he has to escape Mr. B's question. Medicine—so far from Fabiola—has become the complex of forces that puts the young physician in the tunnel and deforms his sense of what he needs to remain alive there. He knows the heart monitoring won't help him; his expertise is irrelevant. He cannot imagine that what could help is communion with the person on the gurney, who at that moment is not so much his patient as his guest and fellow-traveler. I attribute the demoralization to medicine because Peschel acts like too many other physicians in medical stories.

Anthropologist Robert Hahn, in his ethnography of medical culture, describes the work of an internal medical specialist whom he calls Barry Siegler. Siegler explains to Hahn why he cut off his questions to a certain patient. "And I, you know, I've . . . there are a lot of things I didn't even get into with her. I'm just damned afraid of opening a Pandora's, and I wouldn't know how the hell to put the lid back on, so I, I just circumvented a lot of areas." [11] It's easy to imagine that someone like Siegler taught Peschel, who then hears Mr. B's question "opening a Pandora's." Peschel wants to escape a situation that he may not know how "to put the lid back on." The breakdown of dialogue is twofold: for the patients who have the lid kept on what they may need to say, and for the professionals who spend their lives keeping lids on other people.

Hahn presents Barry Siegler as in most respects an exemplary physician whose patients are grateful to have him as their doctor. Good institutional, professional rationales could be offered for his cutting off questions to his patient—and it makes some difference that he cuts off his own questions to his patient, not that he tries to escape questions she has asked him. But Siegler keeps a lid on recognizing what life is like for his patient who is living *in* the Pandora's box. His refusal to ask questions that he knows need to be asked—and he avoids asking them precisely because he knows they open significant issues—is a functional problem insofar as it affects what Komesaroff calls the medical need "to establish common ground on which mutual decisions can be taken." [12] But the problem is also moral: like any withdrawal from dialogue, Siegler's circumventing demoralizes both physician and patient.

One increment past Barry Siegler on the demoralization scale is a physician, "Bill Smith," quoted by sociologist Charles Bosk in his ethnography of genetics counseling in pediatric hospitals. Bosk asks

Smith "how he came to grips with all the 'accidents' or 'mistakes' that he saw." Smith replies:

What you have to do is this, Bosk. When you get up in the morning, pretend your car is a spaceship. Tell yourself you are going to visit another planet. You say, "on that planet terrible things happen, but they don't happen on my planet. They only happen on that planet I take my spaceship to each morning."[13]

Like Barry Siegler, Bill Smith is neither a bad person nor a bad doctor. He is a demoralized person who acts in ways that expand that demoralization, and he lacks the moral imagination to act differently. Bakhtin writes, obliquely but provocatively, of "the complex problem of humiliation and the humiliated."[14] Bill Smith's spaceship expresses the humiliation of someone who cannot take full responsibility for who he is and how he acts. Moreover, we can easily imagine that his patients feel humiliated by their need to be in this place where "terrible things happen." Generosity is the opposite of this humiliation of feeling trapped in a situation you did not create and cannot control. Generosity asserts its own choice, trusting the promise that if you choose for the other, you will make your own life possible.

Physician Rachel Remen describes one way the "spaceship" evasion can end, recalling a retirement dinner she attended early in her career. After the physician being honored had given a talk that Remen describes as "an intellectual *tour de force*" and received a standing ovation, a group of medical students gathers around him.

One of our number asked him if he had any words for us now at the beginning of our careers, anything he thought we should know. He hesitated. But then he told us that despite his professional success and recognition he felt he knew nothing more about life now than he had at the beginning. That he was no wiser. His face became withdrawn, even sad. "It has slipped through my fingers," he said.

None of us knew what he meant.[15]

Stories by physicians who recognize their demoralization early in their careers, and how they seek ways to avoid having their lives and work slip through their fingers, will be told in chapter 4.

How is Mr. B demoralized by his young physician's nonresponse to his obvious question? Mr. B has had his second heart attack within a year. He sees what he and Peschel see in the tunnel. Next, any discussion of what they have seen is, in Barry Siegler's phrase, circumvented.

What they have seen is an evocative image of death—one can't get much more evocative than a sheet-covered corpse within touching distance. The physician who was with him when they confronted this image refuses to acknowledge what they share as common experience.

Philosopher Hilde Lindemann Nelson explores the dark side of the centrality of dialogue in sustaining human selves: precisely because people realize themselves through dialogue with others, others can block that realization. Nelson argues that being fully human requires "the ability to reveal through [one's] actions who [one] is as a person."[16] She calls this revealing "normative self-disclosure."[17] Moral moments, then, are moments of normative self-disclosure. In these moments, like it or not, what we do reveals who we are: the values we uphold and how well we hold them up are evident to ourselves and to others. As we see others react to this self-disclosure, we know ourselves. Curiously, Peschel says nothing about how Mr. B reacted to Peschel's truncated response to the question of what happened in the tunnel. Barry Siegler says nothing about his patient's response to having her questions circumvented. Normative self-disclosure has slipped through their fingers, as Remen's senior physician says at his retirement dinner. He realizes what he has lost.

Normative self-disclosure requires dialogue: the person who we see ourselves revealed to be is seen most fully in others' responses to us. Yet what dialogue enables, refusal of dialogue can deny. This self-disclosure that dialogue makes possible can be impeded when some people refuse to accept others as partners in dialogue.

Much of Nelson's book describes the social conditions that render groups of people unable to perform morally revealing action. She shows the damage those conditions inflict on the identities of members of those groups. Principal among these damaging conditions is others' unwillingness to hear stories in which storytellers place their actions within worthy, significant moral frameworks. Those who block normative self-disclosure in this way tell stories that treat others' actions as indicative of a less than fully mature human consciousness. People treated in this way develop what Nelson calls an "oppressive identity" (27); they are oppressed because their identity is rendered oppressive to them. Oppressive identities are humiliated, in Bakhtin's terms. They are humiliated before they have acted—before the story has even begun—because they have internalized other people's stories about who they can and cannot be. Medical patients acquire oppressive identities when others cut off their telling of stories. In these stories, halting and broken as they often sound, people living disrupted lives seek to place their experience within significant moral frameworks.[18]

If Mr. B could engage in a genuine dialogue about what happened in the tunnel, he might be able to reveal himself as someone who encounters the image of death, under the worst possible circumstances, and survives—he lives to tell the tale. His experience in the tunnel could reveal him to be a kind of hero who passes through the Underworld and returns. But that self-revealing would require a witness. The young Peschel refuses to be a witness in whose presence Mr. B might reveal himself in an empowered identity. Peschel does not simply refuse to talk to Mr. B, he refuses to *recognize* him.

Philosopher Charles Taylor provides an influential statement of the damage people suffer from others' nonrecognition:

> Our identity is partly shaped by recognition, or its absence, often by *mis*recognition of others, so that a person or group of people can suffer real damage, real distortion, if the people or society around them mirror back to them a confining or demeaning or contemptible picture of themselves. Nonrecognition or misrecognition can inflict harm, can be a form of oppression, imprisoning someone in a false, distorted, and reduced mode of being.[19]

In a less frequently quoted passage, Taylor extends the dialogical perspective further: "If some of the things I value most are accessible to me only in relation to the person I love, then she becomes integral to my identity." Taylor discusses how some people might find such dependence to be a limitation, but we have no choice. Taylor argues—following Bakhtin—that humans are able to exist only in relation to other lives. Even solitary lives—the artist or hermit—aspire "to a kind of dialogicality." This tortured word, *dialogicality,* makes the point that there is always an interlocutor: "My own identity crucially depends on my dialogical relations with others" (34).

We return to Nelson's observation that dialogical relations are often distorted in the unequal social distribution of resources each person has available to tell his or her story. These resources include listeners, witnesses, who are willing to recognize the story's significant moral framework. The physician's postural superiority over Mr. B as they go through the tunnel is a fine metaphor for the medical responsibility not only to diagnose and treat patients' diseases but also to witness patients' attempts to understand themselves as morally responsible persons, despite their dependence.[20] There are, certainly, medical moments to act rather than talk: Mr. B's initial admission to the emergency room might be such a moment. But "The Tunnel" describes two moments, in the tunnel and later in Mr. B's room, when action is neither possible nor required; only witness is possible. The failure to offer witness perpetuates everyone's demoralization.

If the stakes on what happens in the tunnel are high for medical hosts and guests, what are the stakes for the society of which the tunnel is part? Jerome wrote about Fabiola because her example set a standard for what he wanted to establish as Christian behavior. The actual help she provided was less important than her symbolic value for upholding the moral responsibility to care for the sick. Contemporary debates about the provision of medical care—who will receive what level of care at whose expense—are venues for working out the limits of moral obligation in a society: who owes what to whom, what can be purchased and what must be forgone if the price cannot be paid, and whose lives have what value under what conditions. In election slogans and mass media advertising, claims about medicine are stand-ins for more expansive visions of social relationships and what obligations these entail.

What happens in medical settings, such as Mr. B's room, both reflects values and expectations in society as a whole, and affects the continuing development of those values. Medical moral moments reflect and affect social expectations of what ought to happen—what's the best that can happen, and what's the minimum that should happen— in other moral moments. When medicine is lost in the tunnel, so is society as a whole. More than workers in any other sphere—except possibly education—medical workers have the responsibility to be hosts, not just providers. Their actions can positively affect social expectations. Medical generosity can show society ways out of the tunnel.

REMORALIZATION IN PRACTICE

"The Tunnel" shows the subtlety of demoralization. What happens is not material for a case study in bioethics; no breach of professional conduct occurs. Peschel the author feels no need to apologize for how he treated Mr. B, and I wonder how many senior physicians would have felt any need to take the young resident aside and suggest he could have acted better. Mr. B's expectations for dialogue with his physicians might have been so low that he shrugged off his physician's unwillingness to respond to his question—and set his future expectations still lower. It takes so little to demoralize—a missed opportunity for dialogue here, a silence there—and generosity often requires little. This book is concerned with getting out of the tunnel, and two stories of how generosity can be renewed set that agenda.

The first story is from the illness narrative of cyclist Lance Armstrong, multiple winner of the Tour de France. Armstrong had testicular cancer that had metastasized as far as his brain. His treatment was successful, and his story suggests that success was not only physical but moral as well:

Shortly before I received my final dose of VIP [chemotherapy], Craig Nichols [Armstrong's oncologist] came by to see me. He wanted to talk about the larger implications of cancer. He wanted to talk about the "obligations of the cured."

It was a subject I had become deeply immersed in. I had said to Nichols and to LaTrice [his nurse] many times over the last three months, "People need to know about this." As I went through therapy, I felt increasing companionship with my fellow patients. . . .

Now I asked about other people. I was startled to read that eight million Americans were living with some form of cancer; how could I possibly feel like mine was an isolated problem? "Can you believe how many people have this?" I asked LaTrice.

"You've changed," she said approvingly. "You're going global." [21]

Armstrong's physician and nurse do what Lammers calls for: they teach their patient something about the limits of medicine as a discipline, and they offer him a moral agenda that begins where medicine currently stops. Their care goes beyond eradicating cancer in Armstrong's body; they care about what sort of moral person he will become through the experience of cancer. They take seriously how they can help him to think beyond the person he has been. They seek to remoralize him. I imagine that if either were asked, he or she would say that this remoralization work is essential to who they are as professionals and as people. [22]

The second remoralization story is my own. [23] During the period leading up to my diagnosis with testicular cancer I underwent a not very skillful bone marrow extraction. As the last part of that procedure some blood had to be drawn, so the physicians departed and a technician came into my room. She was a woman in late middle age, with a sort of rail-thin, weathered look I associate with people who have grown up on the prairies. At least that's what she's become in my memory; I wonder sometimes if I dreamed her.

As this technician went about her work I remarked how skillful she was compared to some other technicians who had been less successful drawing blood from me. She responded by giving me a short lecture on the specific conditions in which I had the right to refuse access to my body: when I could and should tell a technician to quit puncturing me while searching for a vein. She then said something that elevated our encounter to a wholly different plane of significance.

"Remember," she cautioned me, "everyone who touches you affects your healing." In retrospect I hear those words as the first expression of what I eventually realized, and what Armstrong is realizing in the story he tells. I had been thinking that my task was to get to the end of treatment. I suddenly realized my real task would begin once my cancer treatment ended. Then I would have to reassemble a life that would have been touched in so many ways, often by people who seemed indifferent to my healing. Those touches demoralized me. My problem was finding the right touches I needed for healing, and then, eventually, finding others whom I, in turn, might touch as part of their healing.

I do not know how many other medical professionals put themselves out for me in ways I scarcely recognized, but that technician is the one who drew me into a *relation of care*—because care can only be a relationship, a dialogue not only of words but of touch.[24] She found a way to express the recognition that she was not only extracting blood as part of a diagnostic procedure. As a result of how she touched me, she was affecting who I was. Blood drawn in the context of what this woman—whose name I will always regret not learning—said about touching and being touched becomes resonant with all the connotations it derives from being life's fundamental substance, a substance that can be given.

Institutional medicine provides multiple alibis for not entering into relations of care. There are so many good, "managed" reasons for truncating care, for circumventing other people, to use the term that

Hahn reports Barry Siegler using. All these reasons are real in the sense that they reflect the actual demands of medical practice. But these reasons are also unreal, because in the interpersonal moment of practicing medicine, anyone can act differently. The serious question is whether any of the reasons for truncating and circumventing are *good* reasons. Do they create a medical practice that can be a template for the relations of care we want to have prevail in a moral society? Or do they reflect medicine's treatment of its patients as what philosopher Martin Heidegger, in a seminal critique of modern technology, describes as "object[s] on call for inspection."[25] Heidegger uses the medical clinic as an example of a technology that transforms its patients (and its professional workers) into objects for inspection, "subordinate to the orderability" of the clinic (299).

Medical practice reflects both social and personal decisions. Society sets up institutions that determine access to the tools of treatment: which services will be reimbursed at what level, how many operating rooms and diagnostic machines are made available to whom and in what order of preference, which pharmaceuticals are available at what price, and so on. It is a truism that systems of medical treatment and care require reform. The risk is that reforms will be determined by rationales of economic efficiency uninformed by underlying values. But only values can guide how we determine what it is that services are supposed to be efficient at creating.[26] What counts as efficiency depends on what kind of relationships people want between themselves and others, or between themselves and different gradations of others. Do we want to be providers and consumers or to be hosts and guests? In an age when efficiency most often means lowest unit cost, honorable attempts to bring better care to more people may inadvertently increase what Heidegger identified as subordination to orderability.[27] Reform can increase medical demoralization rather than create conditions that facilitate generosity.

When hosts and guests meet face to face, each must decide in that moral moment who he or she will be in relationship to the other. Somewhere in the black hole of my piles of old journals is a speech given by Vaclav Havel soon after he became president of what was then a unified Czechoslovakia.[28] Havel talked to the Czech people about how decades of communist imperialism had demoralized them, leaving them with what Nelson calls an oppressive identity. Under communism, people were unable to see their moral selves revealed in their actions; instead they could see themselves only as actors in a story imposed on them from elsewhere. That oppressive identity, Havel told them, would not be easily set aside. Nor could it be set aside by reform from above, because part of the oppressive story had been that actions were determined by structures imposed from above. People had to reform themselves. Havel called on them to enact their own stories that would reveal the moral frameworks in which they choose to live. No other person, least of all any person in authority, could create those stories for them.

Havel realized that the success of any institutional reform in postcommunist Czechoslovakia depended on individual moral work. People had to effect their own remoralization in the ways they did their work and related to others. He exhorted his listeners to act in ways that revealed identities for which they took full responsibility. Government would carry out its work of reforming old corruptions. But moral identity would not come about because institutions were reformed, nor could it wait for that reform.

When I read Havel I thought of contemporary health care and its perpetual promises of institutional reform. As medicine expands its capabilities—especially the costly capacity to keep more people alive, longer, with more debilitating conditions—institutional reform will always be a work in progress. No one should have any illusions about the capacity of institutional reform to bring about a renewal of generosity. It's the reverse: personal acts of generosity have the potential to affect the values that determine what goals are sought by reform. In clinics, at the bedside where it counts, a health care system is people touching each other. Everyone who touches anyone affects that person's healing, and affects the further demoralization of medicine— or its remoralization. In the moral moment of that touch, there is no system.

CHAPTER TWO

The Dialogical Stoic

S AM Crane turns to the ancient Chinese *Book of Changes* for guidance on how he should live after the birth of his disabled son, Aidan. Aidan's brain lacks the tissue bridging the cerebral hemispheres, a condition that can have a range of effects. For Aidan it means being quadriplegic, blind, and incapable of speech. He will always wear diapers; he will never use signs or words to communicate. Crane's story tells how he learns to be a father to Aidan, becoming comfortable meeting needs he never expected having to confront.

When faced with such devastation, you call upon whatever personal resources you have, whatever will work to keep you afloat. For some, it may be the comfort of family, for others the transcendence of religion or the rationality of science. Not for me. . . . When in trouble, I looked elsewhere for answers and support. One alternative was the Book of Changes.

SAM CRANE

⌘

Crane is a professor of Asian studies, so it's not surprising he finds a resource in ancient Chinese wisdom: first the *I Ching* or *Book of Changes,* and later the writing of Chuang Tzu and Lao Tzu. Other people's writing about their illnesses, including my own, uses these sages to make sense of what was happening to them, to give their suffering meaning, and to articulate what can seem impossible to express.[1] I could have looked to Taoist and Zen writings to give greater resonance to the stories of illness in this book, and perhaps I will write that book someday. But as I started writing, those sages remained outside my study. Who walked in, sat down, and had to be written about was the Dialogical Stoic.

When I was in graduate school Carlos Castaneda's anthropological fiction (or was it? that was the question) expressed the not-so-secret fantasy of many young people.[2] Castaneda, a graduate student in anthropology, goes into the Mexican desert to do research and meets the Yaqui sorcerer don Juan. The sorcerer imparts all manner of wisdom, including how to do neat things like walk up walls, fly through canyons, and project a double of himself, to fill in at his less interesting appointments. We'd all like to meet a don Juan. If I've given that up, the closest I can get is the Dialogical Stoic, who wears the gray wool cloak of an ancient Roman, has a face that seems Russian with its trace of pain, and speaks with a French accent.

If the Dialogical Stoic were to come to life as a single being, she would sound like a stand-up comic's version of multiple personality disorder. My interest is not to sort out the different voices of the Dialogical Stoic. As I wrote in the introduction, the trope of a persona is a way to avoid creating an ism. To borrow the phrasing of Lance Armstrong's title, it's not about the Dialogical Stoic, any more than Sam Crane writes a book about the ancient Chinese sages. At a time when Crane was sinking, he could use fragments from the sages to make a figurative raft to keep himself afloat. The Dialogical Stoic is such a raft.

The Chinese sages show Crane what he can learn from Aidan. The sages provide a measure of *what counts*. They add resonance to Crane's personal story, connecting his struggles and discoveries to perennial human attempts to understand how to live. The sages become Crane's *reflecting team*, a practice I discussed in the introduction. They mirror his experiences and insights in a different language; they suggest which ways of understanding and acting he should cultivate and which he should avoid. My reflecting team is the Dialogical Stoic, which brings together, but does not unify, two traditions of thought that have indispensable relevance for ill people and those who care for them.

I have already quoted the Stoic philosopher Marcus Aurelius to provide a reflection that moves the introduction toward the moral task of medicine. Chapter 1 talks about dialogue and Mikhail Bakhtin. This chapter's more extended introduction of Stoicism and dialogical thought begins with two reflections on illness and a story of care. The first is from my own experience of illness, and the second returns to Sam Crane to describe the experience of giving care.

I was seriously ill more than fifteen years ago. Some memories of this time remain vivid and others merge into patterns. Two patterns that organize my memories are time spent alone—hours when other people were engaged in the tasks that healthy people spend their time

on, while I was too sick to do anything but lay there—and time spent
with people who were willing to listen to me as I worked toward a story
that made sense of my life with illness.

The time spent alone required me to cultivate an inner dialogue—
an imagination of myself that I could live with, a literal expression
given the condition I was in. During times alone, the only choice that
was mine to make was how I imagined myself. Everything else—from
my body outward—was beyond my control. These times recalled the
Stoic lesson that what matters is how you regard your situation, the
sense you choose to make of it. The Stoic asks: who are you choosing
to be, regardless of where you find yourself, and is that your best
choice?

The times when I was with other people fed my developing realization of how dependent I was on their imaginations of me. I knew myself through these others. I experienced what Bakhtin says in the epigraph to chapter 1: I had no internal sovereignty; I existed only on the
boundary that is communion with others. Fifteen years ago I had no
words to name these two times; now I call them Stoic and dialogical.
Those labels help sort out what is possible, and what is required, in different moments of illness. They console suffering, and part of their
consolation is to challenge how we suffer. Their challenges are forms
of consolation because they promise the suffering person that we are
still actively shaping our life; they offer a purpose. If mixing Stoicism
with dialogical theory is a philosophical oxymoron, this mix fits the
experience of someone living in deep illness. Like Sam Crane in the
epigraph to this chapter, I called on whatever would keep me afloat.

I turn from the experience of illness to the experience of offering
care. One of Sam Crane's stories of caring for Aidan illustrates the
complementary necessity of Stoicism and dialogue. Crane expresses
his communion with Aidan—the physical intimacy is tangible. He is
also engaging in a form of Stoic spiritual exercise. He controls his attention to the reality outside himself, and he shapes how he understands his relation to this reality.

Every morning, before taking him into the social world of school, I wash Aidan.
We do this while he is still in bed, lying straight on his back. Starting with his
face, I slip my left hand under his head to steady it and speak to him, alerting
him to the coming shock of dampness on his brow. Even with my spoken intro-

duction, the first swipes of the warm washcloth invariably startle him. He widens
his eyes in reaction to the wet assault. I carefully rub under and behind his ears,
working toward his eyes to cleanse away the sleep from their inner corners. Soap
comes next, soap on cheeks and forehead and chin, soap to dissolve the dirt from
his smooth skin.[3]

Crane's description of washing Aidan continues for another page and a
half. The writing requires this length of detail to approximate real time
so the reader can experience the scene as Crane experiences it. Crane
calls upon the reader to stay with him, just as he stays with Aidan: seeing what is there and doing what has to be done. Crane knows himself
not as someone who accomplishes the task of washing Aidan, but as
someone who brings the dignity and comfort of being clean to his son,
always recognizing him as a person: "I slip my left hand under his head
to steady it and speak to him, alerting him to the coming shock of
dampness." This is generosity, a scene Fabiola would smile on.

The Dialogical Stoic may be a philosophical oxymoron, but it can be
an experiential reality.

Marcus's Universal Stoicism

My grandmother gave me my first copy of Marcus Aurelius's *Meditations* on my fifteenth birthday. It's now fragile; a beautifully illustrated, limited edition that she had received as a wedding present in
1913. I was fortunate to discover Marcus through a gift; a chance encounter would be next best. Phillip Simmons describes such an encounter in the meditations he wrote while he was living with amy-
otrophic lateral sclerosis (ALS), or motor neuron disease.[4] He came
upon a leather-bound copy of Marcus among some books that his wife,
an artist, was about to use as "sculptural materials to be hacked,
drilled, sawed, lacquered, slathered in plaster and cast in bronze" (18).
Simmons saved this copy of Marcus to be read instead of hacked, and
he wrote about how that reading consoled him.

Marcus's writing has a history of being saved from the scrap heap,
a curiosity that may enhance its interest to those who live with illness
and disability. The classicist Pierre Hadot, on whose scholarship I am
most dependent, writes that "the greatest uncertainty often reigns"
as to whether the text we now have is what Marcus wrote.[5] The leading British scholar of Marcus's work, R. B. Rutherford, notes that the

Meditations—untitled by Marcus himself and probably not intended for others' reading—survived as a single copy, written by Marcus himself or by a scribe and preserved by Marcus's family or a secretary. The first references to the book appear several hundred years after Marcus died in A.D. 180. A number of manuscripts from late antiquity contain extracts of his writing, just as he includes extracts of other philosophers, notably Heraclitus. The first printed version of *Meditations* was in 1559, based on one of two manuscripts that then existed. Rutherford states that the reader can feel "fairly confident" at finding in contemporary texts "at least a fair reflection" of what Marcus wrote, which to a nonclassicist seems faint reassurance.[6] No one knows how often Marcus's writing was copied by hand before the earliest manuscripts that still exist, and what errors and changes were introduced. This history of textual uncertainty enhances the pleasure and value that readers like Simmons find in Marcus, for living with illness is about incorporating contingent interventions.

Not only is the text uncertain. Marcus wrote in Greek, and he sounds very different in different translations. George Long's 1862 translation is the one my grandmother gave me. It endows or burdens Marcus with Victorian eloquence: long-winded, but with lovely turns of phrase. A. S. L. Farquharson, a soldier as well as a classics teacher, died in 1942, and his translation was published two years later; the current edition is corrected by Rutherford. Farquharson's Marcus sounds to me like an aphorist, speaking from some height to a reader below. Marcus typically phrases his thoughts in the second-person "you." More recent translations emphasize him speaking to himself, exhorting himself to live as he ought to. In Long's and Farquharson's translations, "you" seems addressed to the reader. Marcus sounds like one who already knows and is passing on his accumulated wisdom.

My most recent rediscovery of Marcus is through the translation by classicist Gregory Hays. Hays's lean, spare tone is appropriate to the spirit of moderation Marcus strives for in his life. The tone of struggle and search predominates over assertion. Hays's Marcus, like the recent translations by Pierre Hadot—translated from Hadot's French into English—use exclamation marks to emphasize the self-exhortation of writing as a spiritual exercise.[7] Marcus is not offering his wisdom to posterity but using writing as a means to train himself to live like a Stoic, before it's too late.[8]

I dwell on Marcus's questionable texts and his divergent translations to emphasize what readers like Simmons realize intuitively. Each
reader can discover—not invent, but discover—his or her own Marcus. His writing adapts itself to the reader's need and interest. Hays, in
his introduction to his translation, observes that Marcus has always
been more popular with lay readers than with professional classicists
(xlix). He quotes one such reader, the American memoirist William
Alexander Percy, writing of "the unassailable wintry kingdom of Marcus Aurelius. . . . It is not outside, but within, and when all is lost, it
stands fast" (xlix–l). Percy catches Marcus's uncanny ability to speak
to a reader like a voice from within (and if the voice of one translation
does not speak to you, try another), and Marcus's attraction to those
who seek to stand fast when all is lost.

Phillip Simmons died soon after *Learning to Fall* was published.
Marcus affirms his discovery that standing fast, in Percy's phrase, can
mean learning to fall, a practical necessity for a man with degenerative
muscle disease. Simmons feigns to be initially puzzled by his attraction to Marcus:

> To most of us stoicism means stuffing our feelings, shunning the pleasures of the
> flesh, and refusing to exercise our constitutional right to feel sorry for ourselves
> in public. So you may wonder what odd and possibly masochistic impulse had me
> wanting to write about Marcus Aurelius Antoninus, the Roman emperor and
> Stoic.[9]

Here are my own reasons why ill and disabled people, and those
who care for them, can find consolation in Marcus's Stoicism. Marcus
offers a practical, applied way of living. He was not concerned with
constructing an abstract theory of ethics; he wrote in order to *act well*
in his everyday life.[10] In the first book of the *Meditations*, which is differently presented than what follows, Marcus thanks specific family
members, patrons, friends, and teachers for what each has taught him.
His thanks to his philosophy teacher Rusticus is: "To have had some
idea of the need I had to straighten out my moral condition" (i.7). The
passage summarizes Hadot's argument that for Marcus and others of
his time, to be a philosopher was not to aspire to make a scholarly contribution to some body of theoretical knowledge, but rather to live life
according to certain principles of continual self-development.[11] Hays
writes that philosophy "was not merely a subject to write or argue

about, but one that was expected to provide a 'design for living'—a set of rules to live one's life by" (xix). Marcus's thanks to Rusticus continues: "That I did not let myself be dragged into writing treatises on abstract questions," which would be a strange comment from a contemporary philosopher—but for Marcus, being a philosopher does not mean the academic vocation it implies today. When Marcus thanks another teacher, Diognetus, for having taught him "to practice philosophy" (i.6), to *practice* means working daily to change his habits and way of living.

Marcus writes to correct how he perceives his life and his place in life as a whole, because action begins in correct perception. He writes not to discover anything new, but to remind himself to put into practice what he has learned. His constant message is: this is what you need to remember, if you are serious about wanting to live as humans have the capacity to live and are supposed to live. Readers like William Percy or Phillip Simmons use Marcus to help themselves remember how they ought to live.

The style of Marcus's *Meditations* appeared to me, when I was fifteen, as random thoughts of particular moments. Hadot demonstrates that Marcus was following a specific plan, laid out by the Stoic tradition, for his continuing training and moral development.[12] I will necessarily simplify the system that Hadot proposes, rendering it in a form relevant to being ill and caring for the ill.

People are most likely to feel called to Stoicism when adversity strikes. Hadot writes of "the blow which sets the inner discourse of the guiding principle in motion" (106); recall Barbara Rosenblum's description, in chapter 1, of receiving a diagnosis of cancer. The biography of Marcus's early life allows for interpretive guesses that he might have suffered some such blow, but these are only guesses. What matters is that his Stoicism is a philosophy for those who encounter suffering and must discover a way to live with it.

The Stoic response to suffering begins with detachment. Simmons is joking in his quip about Stoicism's "shunning all pleasures of the flesh" (after Marcus's wife died, he took a concubine), but Stoicism does cultivate a detached attitude toward the body. The reason for this detachment is based in Stoic theory of perception. Marcus writes (xii.3) that humans are composed of three components: body, vital breath (that animates life), and mind or intellect. Our bodies are ours to take care of, and Marcus praises his adoptive father, Antoninus Pius, for "his willingness to take adequate care of himself" (i.16). But the body's inevitable decline places it among the external things that humans cannot control, just as we cannot control when we will die. Thus among the three components, a person truly is mind, or intellect, intelligence, understanding—the variation between translations suggests that the meaning involves more than we understand by any of these words alone. Mind is not isolated intellect; the mind's capacity for rationality practices on and through the body. In a unified body-mind, mind represents the capacity for choice, and physical body represents what cannot be chosen. Stoicism calls for detaching the thinking capacity, for which you can be responsible, from the body, to which misfortunes occur that you cannot control.

Stoic detachment from the body is not Christian asceticism that shuns pleasures of the flesh because these are sinful. The Stoic seeks *freedom*, and detachment is a practice aimed at freeing yourself from living in fear of what fate may do to your body. For Simmons, the blow of diagnosis brings him to Marcus, whose consolation is that if the body is falling, the mind does not have to fall with it. Learning to fall means accepting that the flesh can fall without injury to what counts about the self: its character, expressed in controlling the perception and understanding of events, and in choosing how to react.

The need to achieve this independence from the body derives from more than anticipation of injury, illness, or age. People in any condition of health need the discipline of gaining control of how our perceptions affect us. Hadot describes the Stoic differentiation between two levels of perception. He quotes Epictetus, a Stoic who influenced Marcus, on the crucial distinction between *representations* and what is translated as *assents*. Representations "throw themselves upon people," who are rendered passive. The *body* responds involuntarily to representations, feeling fear, disgust, desire, or whatever. That feeling is then assumed to be an inherent property of what is represented, and for the Stoics, the error of immediately associating the reality with a judgment is a root cause of human unhappiness and discontent.

Stoic practice begins in understanding that representations "do not depend upon the will, and are not free" (Epictetus, quoted by Hadot, 102). By contrast, what Hadot translates as *assents* are just that: consciously assented to, rather than involuntarily responded to. Assents are "representations [that] are recognized and judged, are voluntary and take place through human freedom" (Hadot, 102).

Gaining freedom from fears about the body requires practicing what Hadot calls the *discipline of assent:* interrupting the body's habitual responses (which even the sage can never extinguish; the effect can only be shortened) and deciding which representations to respond to and how to respond. Hadot presents the Stoic discipline of assent as having four stages; again I will use a diagnosis of illness as an example. First is the *external event;* someone tells Simmons he has ALS. Second is the *representation* of that event. A value judgment is added to the perception of the event, immediately and involuntarily. What *is* is no longer seen as it is, but as good or bad. Barbara Rosenblum's description of her reaction to being diagnosed as having breast cancer depicts the body's involuntary, visceral reaction to the representation. Third, the Stoic interrupts the involuntary response. The representation is heard or seen not as reality itself but as a *discourse* or image. The mind says no to the value judgment, suspends it, and sees only what is, then and there. The diagnosis is understood as words someone says, and *nothing more.* The fourth and final stage is the *assent:* the Stoic separates the external event into those aspects that can be controlled by the mind and those that are external and beyond control. The Stoic assents to be concerned only with what affects his or her moral character.

The discipline of assent replaces the body's involuntary reaction with a reaction that is chosen by the mind. The Stoic mind (again, a translation to be understood warily) is not separated from the body. The mind is *freed to choose* how to understand what is happening to the body. Free, in Simmons's terms, to learn that falling can be all right if you fall without judging the falling. This assent renders Simmons free to live with illness as he can, rather than living according to how someone with ALS is represented. Thus Stoicism anticipates the contemporary disability rights movement, which asserts the freedom to accept oneself as differently abled.

The discipline of assent is a practice for living according to the Stoic conviction that exterior events are not what trouble us; rather we are troubled by our judgments of those events. Both Rosenblum and Simmons die of their diseases, but the Stoic accepts death as what happens to bodies. Disease and death are external in the sense of being beyond our control. What counts is that Rosenblum and Simmons do not allow sickness to determine how they express who they are. They over-come their initial representation of their illness and practice assent: both decide what to allow the disease to mean in their lives. "If you are grieving about some exterior thing, then it is not that thing which is troubling you, but your judgment about that thing," Marcus reminds himself (viii.47).

The discipline of assent, the separation of what can be controlled from what is external, and the freedom that results from suspend-ing judgments are all summarized in Marcus's counterintuitive observation:

> It's the pursuit of these things, and your attempts to avoid them, that leave you in such turmoil. And yet they aren't seeking you out; you are the one seeking them.
>
> Suspend judgment about them. And at once they will lie still, and you will be freed from fleeing and pursuing. (xi.11, Hays trans.)

In chapter 1, the young physician's attempts to avoid the tunnel—at-tempts that lead him to evade his patient's question about what hap-pened there—leave him in turmoil. His disturbance at seeing the fu-neral cortege exemplifies the dangers of being unable to interrupt the body's initial reaction to representations. He does not see what is—a group he cannot make sense of but who are, nonetheless, only people; he projects unnamed fears into what he is seeing. Even when he learns what he saw, he cannot separate what actually was from those fears. He will never "escape" the tunnel (that is, he will never escape his need to escape) until he takes responsibility for his representations, both of the tunnel and of his patient, Mr. B.

Sam Crane's life and narrative is about coming to know Aidan's physical condition as exterior, in a Stoic sense. His story is about changing his perception of Aidan's condition; specifically, how he learns what to allow to trouble him. Crane cannot control Aidan's blindness or his inability to use his hands or legs. That Aidan is unlike other chil-dren is not troubling because it is how Aidan is. Aidan's untreated pain *is* troubling, because that's a medical failure and can be changed. Most illness narratives follow this Stoic plot of learning which judgments to assent to.

Illness—whether one's own or that of a loved one—appears to seek us out, but that's our representation. The difficult wisdom is learning what Marcus says: we seek out the exterior thing by the judgments that we allow to affect how we perceive it. Those unchosen judgments harm something valuable within us.

Hadot emphasizes the idea, prevalent in ancient philosophy, that each person has an indwelling *daimōn*. Marcus is unclear exactly what this interior power or divinity is and how it differs from the mind or intellect. Hadot eventually proposes understanding the *daimōn* as "the absolute value or moral intent and the love of moral good" (124), but these words require more words to define them. If I want to see what the *daimōn* is, I think of Crane washing his son or Simmons learning to fall without judging himself. The *daimōn* is what allows us to express the best part of ourselves, the part that we ought to seek to defend and to expand until it shapes each of our acts. Marcus's greatest concern is to avoid what can corrupt and diminish his *daimōn*.

Simmons's body does deteriorate, and Rosenblum's cancer spreads; they die. Marcus is perhaps most eloquent training himself to prepare to die with as much freedom as possible, without, that is, losing himself to fears and judgments he does not choose. I will condense Marcus's thoughts on death to three, which are all familiar themes in the contemporary therapeutic literature on dying. Familiar, that is, as abstractions; the Stoic point is to *practice* integrating this knowledge into the body's responses. First is Marcus's idea that what is to be feared is not death itself. A worthy fear—a fear that can inform our lives for the good—is fear of never having lived well or fully before we die. Second, preparation for death involves cultivating a certainty that one exists as a very small part of an unthinkably large cosmos. We cannot know the ways of this cosmos, but Marcus insists that it is good. "To love what happens, what was destined. No greater harmony" (vii.57). In recomposing this thought in many variations, Marcus trains himself to believe it.

Marcus's third insight into death is that like any other external event, death itself should not trouble us: "Death: something like birth, a natural mystery, elements that split and recombine. Not an embarrassing thing. Not an offense to reason, or our nature" (Hays, iv.37). Here is the core of Marcus's consolation for the critically ill: know death as dissolving back into the whole from which we came, and from which we may emerge again, in some form. The lyricism of this thought consoles. Marcus is not promising eternal life, but, following Heraclitus, he does propose that endings may be more apparent than real.

Marcus's thoughts on death seem to be those that most attract Phillip Simmons. The copy of the *Meditations* that Simmons rescued from his wife's art studio must have been George Long's translation, with its Victorian phrases sounding like the King James Version of the Bible. Simmons quotes this passage:

> Let it make no difference to thee whether thou art cold or warm, if [i.e., so long as] thou art doing thy duty; and whether thou art drowsy or satisfied with sleep; and whether ill-spoken or praised; and whether dying or doing something else. For it is one of the acts of life, this act by which we die: it is sufficient then in this act also to do well what we have in hand. (vi.2)

Hays presents Marcus in a more terse idiom: "Dying . . . or busy with other assignments" (ellipses in original). This is the line that Simmons values. Simmons was near his death, and Marcus told him not to fear dying but to approach death like another assignment, something to do well. Control representations; choose what to assent to; remain free. Protect the best part of yourself.

Simmons understands that Marcus does not denigrate the flesh. Marcus teaches instead how to achieve freedom from worry about it. Simmons summarizes Marcus's consolation: "The freedom, first, from attachment to the things of this life that don't really matter: fame, material possessions, and even, finally, our own bodies. Acceptance brings the freedom to live fully in the present."[13] This freedom is always available to us, even—especially—when we are dying . . . or doing something else.

Hadot, after all his scholarly emphasis on comprehending the specific philosophical system that underlies Marcus's apparent randomness of thought, imagines a universal or eternal Stoicism that is "one of the fundamental, permanent possibilities of human existence, when people search for wisdom" (310). In the final pages of his monograph on Marcus, Hadot suggests parallels between Marcus and a seventeenth-century Chinese philosopher, Wang-Fou-chic. The more contemporary parallel is to psychiatrist and Holocaust survivor Viktor Frankl, who discovered that even in the Nazi concentration camps, in conditions of the most overt physical brutality,

> [t]here were always choices to make. Every day, every hour, offered the opportunity to make a decision, a decision which determined whether you would or would not submit to those powers which threatened to rob you of your very self,

your inner freedom; which determined whether or not you would become the
plaything of circumstance, renouncing freedom and dignity to become molded
into the form of the typical inmate.[14]

Frankl does not use the language of protecting his *daimōn*, but he
seems to have reached the same understanding of his humanity when
he writes of "this spiritual freedom—which cannot be taken away—
that makes life meaningful and purposeful" (87).

Hadot describes this universal Stoicism as having three core beliefs,
which are each consolations for the ill. First, "no being is alone, but . . .
we are parts of a Whole. . . . The Stoic constantly has his mind on this
Whole." Second, the Stoic "feels absolutely serene, free, and invul-
nerable, insofar as he has become aware that there is no other evil than
moral evil, and that the only thing that counts is the purity of moral
conscience." Within this consolation, I would add the promise that
each of us remains free to protect our *daimōn* from corruption. The
third belief of eternal Stoicism is what Hadot calls "the universal value
of the human person" (311). He claims that Stoicism is the origin of
our contemporary understanding of human rights.

Marcus's promise of individual freedom and his understanding of
that freedom as a challenge pervade Vaclav Havel's speech, discussed in
chapter 1. Havel tells postcommunist Czechs not to wait for government reforms but to act for themselves, on themselves. Marcus constantly reminds himself that what he wants for himself requires only
his assent, and he repeatedly asks himself what he could be waiting for.
Hadot concludes his discussion of universal Stoicism by quoting
Havel's summation of the goal of politics, which could be a translation
of Marcus: "to try and remain in harmony with my conscience and
with my better self" (306).

To understand Stoicism as eternal is not, however, to claim it is
sufficient. When I am ill and alone, subject to all manner of fears, I
would like Marcus's thoughts to be my thoughts. To prepare for illness
I could imagine nothing better than to devise a version of the spiritual
exercise that writing the *Meditations* was for Marcus. But what about
relationships with other people? The Stoic may have a powerful realization of others' rights, but Marcus rarely expresses pleasure in being
with other people. The exemplary family, friends, and teachers to
whom he expresses gratitude in book 1 of the *Meditations* are all dead.

Marcus has a compelling notion of service to others, yet what is he saying about himself when he writes: "And you—on the verge of death—you still refuse to care for them, although you're one of them yourself" (vii.70).

Marcus spent much of his life participating in military campaigns— he died while on campaign—and military images and metaphors fill the *Meditations*. In one of these Marcus advises himself to be "Not a dancer but a wrestler: waiting, poised and dug in, for sudden assaults" (vii.61). He may be referring to the assaults of representations to which he does not wish to assent, but the passage expresses the defensiveness that pervades his writing. If Marcus seems at peace with the whole of the cosmos, he remains guarded with his fellow creatures. Only with the dead does he seem to relax. In his situation, what else could we expect? I can never presume to judge Marcus, the intrigue and brutality of whose world are beyond my imagination. But in my world, I believe that illness and care need more than his Stoicism.

Dialogue and the Hero

The idea of dialogue was introduced in chapter 1 as what is missing in the relationship between Peschel and Mr. B in "The Tunnel." This chapter begins with a dialogue in which Sam Crane washes his son, Aidan, and takes care to speak to the child, who cannot understand the words, lest he shock him with the wet cloth. Crane knows his son as someone whom he affects, and he knows himself as affected by Aidan, who has become part of who Sam Crane is.

The Russian literary critic Mikhail Bakhtin spent his long life developing a moral ideal of human relationships as dialogue. Bakhtin was born in 1895 in Russia, did graduate work in Germany, returned to his native country, and began writing at the time of the Russian Revolution. Bakhtin's life and literary production can be as shadowy as Marcus Aurelius's recopied text. We can be fairly certain that he wrote most of what is attributed to him, but within Bakhtin's circle, pseudonyms were used to evade censorship. Even when his authorship is certain, we can never know what he concealed in tropes chosen to pass the censor. Bakhtin was arrested and during the early 1930s served a sentence as an internal exile, teaching school in Kustani.[15] He lived until 1975, which was remarkable given the political persecution and chronic illness he experienced. His major work was published in the last years of his life, and his writings received international recognition only after his death.[16]

Bakhtin writes about authors and their characters; the dialogical relationship as he depicts it is between author and hero, and between the characters themselves. As I stated earlier, when I am ill and alone, I would like Marcus's thoughts to be mine. However, when I am ill and among others, I would want to be part of the relationships of Bakhtinian dialogue. First, I hope for physicians and nurses who act toward me as Bakhtin describes Dostoevsky as author acting toward his characters. Simon Dentith summarizes Bakhtin's insight that Dostoevsky's novels "grant the voices of the main characters as much authority as the narrator's voice, which indeed engages in active dialogue with the characters' voices."[17] Dostoevsky "speaks not about a character, but with him," Bakhtin writes.[18] This difference between speaking *about* and speaking *with* was what I argued that the young physician in "The Tunnel" fails to understand. The moral demand of dialogue is that each grant equal authority to the other's voice. Committing yourself to dialogue with people is more than recognizing their inherent dignity and defending their rights; it's being willing to allow their voice to count as much as yours.

Bakhtin idealizes dialogue as each person having the will and capacity to see the situation, and to see themselves, "in all the mirrors of other people's consciousnesses"; the dialogical hero "knows all the possible refractions of his image in those mirrors" (53). My ideal clinic is where each participant—medical workers, patients, volunteers, and friends—sees what is happening in all the possible refractions of the mirrors of one another's perceptions. Each is constantly asking: what does this look like to *them*, from where they are?

Here we reach the practical impossibility of dialogical thought and ethics. None of us can know *all* the mirrors of other people's consciousnesses and see ourselves refracted in all those mirrors, all the time. Perfection can be a useful goal, however, even if it is never achieved. We can seek to expand how many of the possible refractions we see, and expand how thoroughly our consciousness is pervaded by what we see in these mirrors. We can keep in mind that our most conspicuous moral failures result from not looking at ourselves in the mirrors of enough other consciousnesses. We can keep the question before us: what do they think about how I am imagining them? And we can believe that what they think matters.

The imperative of our own agenda—what patients' fears impose on them, and what physicians' and nurses' expertise and experience compels them to believe is necessary—has the kind of physical effect on us that Stoicism attributes to external representations. We feel our needs and purposes are reality, and then we believe ourselves justified in acting on this reality. Bakhtin's general designation for this condition is *monologue:* one voice believing that it alone is sufficient. Just as Stoics train themselves to interrupt the effect that external representations have on them, stripping these representations of their judgments in order to see what is and nothing more, so dialogical thinkers interrupt the monological pursuit of their own purposes and self-perceptions. A dialogical ethic calls us to imagine what we look like—acting as we are—to the people around us, and grant those perceptions equal validity.

Bakhtin, no less than Marcus, undertakes remaking how he sees life and human relationships. "Interrogate yourself," Marcus writes, "to find out what inhabits your so-called mind and what kind of soul you have now" (v.11). Bakhtin interrogates Dostoevsky to find the model of a new kind of soul, created and sustained in dialogue. In learning to read Dostoevsky as he does, he works on his own mind and soul. Literary criticism becomes spiritual exercise, and that exercise can inform illness and medicine.

Dostoevsky's creative method, or the method Bakhtin attributes to him, becomes a model of moral life:

> At the center of Dostoevsky's creative work there stands, in place of the relationship of a single cognizant and judging "I" to the world, the problem of the interrelationship of all these cognizant and judging "I's" to one another. (99–100)

The moral moment occurs when we who imagine ourselves as "a single cognizant and judging 'I'" must decide whether to give equal weight to the other cognizant and knowing I's around us. We acknowledge, or we do not acknowledge, that the very possibility of our self and thoughts has always depended on others. We enter into dialogue, or not.

For Bakhtin there is no choice except to enter into dialogue, because the self has its origin and its ongoing existence only in that realm. His brief developmental history of a human being is worth quoting, because it is the foundation of the dialogical perspective:

> Everything that pertains to me enters my consciousness, beginning with my name, from the external world through the mouths of others (my mother, and so

forth), with their intonation, in their emotional and value-assigning tonality. I realize myself initially through others: from them I receive words, forms, and tonalities for the formation of my initial idea of myself. The elements of infantilism in self-awareness ("Could mama really love such a . . . ") sometimes remain until the end of life (perception and the idea of one's self, one's body, face, and past in tender tones). Just as the body is formed initially in the mother's womb (body), a person's consciousness awakens wrapped in another's consciousness.[19]

To be "wrapped in another's consciousness" involves a tension that seems at the core of Bakhtin's dialogical understanding of how humans relate to each other. One side of this tension is what he calls "nonself-sufficiency."[20] The boundaries of our selves are more permeable than real: the hero's "words about himself are structured under the continuous influence of someone else's words about him" (207). As Bakhtin writes in the passage quoted as the epigraph to chapter 1, we have no internal sovereignty as individuals; we exist only on the boundary with others. "Not that which takes place within," Bakhtin declares, "but that which takes place on the boundary between one's own and someone else's consciousness, on the threshold" (287).

In tension with nonself-sufficiency, Bakhtin makes a clear demand that one consciousness not lapse into merging with others. Katrina Clark and Michael Holquist summarize this requirement to sustain difference:

The way in which I create myself is by means of a quest: I go out to the other in order to come back with a self. I "live into" an other's consciousness; I see the world through that other's eyes. But I must never completely meld with that version of things, for the more successfully I do, the more I will fall prey to the limitation of the other's horizon. A complete fusion . . . even were it possible, would preclude the difference required by dialogue.[21]

Sustaining the difference that dialogue requires means never speaking "finalizing words" about another; such words would "debase the human being-personality" (296). No word can ever be final because anyone can choose to act differently. The unfinalizability of the literary character—or the medical patient—is what requires the author or physician to speak *with* him, not *about* him. Only a finalized character could be spoken about, and to speak about a character is to finalize him. Hosts never finalize guests; they remain open to whoever the guest may become.

If nonself-sufficiency recognizes our immersion in our social milieu, unfinalizability recognizes that milieu is not destiny for any person, any more than personal history is destiny. The others whose voices are in our voice, through whose eyes we see ourselves, do not determine us. As Clark and Holquist write, I go out to the other in order to come back with a self that retains its own horizons. The objective of going out is not to be limited by my own horizons; the object of return is not to exchange my own limitations for those of someone else.

"To be means to communicate dialogically," Bakhtin writes. "When the dialogue ends, everything ends."[22] This statement recalls the epigraph of chapter 1, in which Bakhtin describes "absolute death" as "the state of being unheard, unrecognized, unremembered." Bakhtin must have lived with the fear that his writings would remain unpublished and eventually be lost; the fear that as a result of Stalinist oppression, he might die unheard, unrecognized, unremembered. By choosing to continue to write, despite censorship and illness, he offers witness to the possibility of resisting the "absolute death" he describes. Bakhtin, censored and persecuted, idealizes dialogue that makes communion with the other its measure of existence; as if in response to Marcus's self-exhortation, he shows what kind of soul he has.

However singular Bakhtin's biography, he is not alone in recognizing that beyond the linguistic construction of the separate "I," no firm boundary separates self and other. At the beginning of the twentieth century, this idea was explored by pragmatists (William James, George Herbert Mead); in midcentury it was developed in theology (Martin Buber), phenomenology (Maurice Merleau-Ponty), and hermeneutics (Martin Heidegger, Hans-Georg Gadamer). Two contemporary exponents of the dialogical perspective were discussed in chapter 1: Charles Taylor, whose work integrates Bakhtin within a broad philosophical tradition, and Hilde Nelson, whose work is part of a rich literature of feminist relational ethics.

But as I wrote in the introduction, a reflecting team must limit its number of voices, lest the members begin to discuss their own differences. As I restricted Stoicism to Marcus Aurelius, despite all that Epictetus, Cicero, Seneca, and others might contribute, so I limit dialogical thought to Bakhtin and Emmanuel Levinas. If justification of these two is required, it is that the life and thought of each was formed by his direct encounter with one of the two greatest horrors of the twentieth century: for Bakhtin, Stalinism, and for Levinas, the Holocaust.

Levinas was born in Lithuania in 1906, studied philosophy in Germany in the 1930s, and was a student of the young, charismatic Martin Heidegger. He then began an academic career in Paris. During World War II Levinas served as an interpreter in the French army and spent most of the war as a German prisoner. Remarkably, the Nazis honored the Geneva convention with respect to their Jewish prisoners of war. Levinas did outdoor manual labor, received Red Cross packages, and continued reading philosophy. After the war he learned that his entire family, except his wife and daughter, had been killed in Nazi camps. His wife and daughter had been helped by friends and eventually hidden by French Catholic nuns; Levinas later recalled that assistance as one of his paradigms of moral generosity. His important philosophical work was written fairly late in his career, but he had a long life, dying in 1996.[23] In his brief autobiographical essay "Signature," written in the third person, Levinas follows a capsule history of his career with a sentence that sounds like his own epitaph: "It is dominated by the presentiment and the memory of the Nazi horror."[24]

Levinas's core dictum is that "all men are responsible for one another" (169), an idea that he, like Bakhtin, finds most clearly expressed in Dostoevsky. How Levinas understands this responsibility is best exemplified in the trope of the *face*. In this Levinas does not mean some arrangement of eyes, nose, and mouth. To see the other's face is to recognize that other as needing me and to feel chosen in the primacy of my obligation to meet that need. Levinas explains:

I define face precisely by these traits beyond vision or confusion with the vision of the face. One can say once more: the face . . . is like a being's exposure to death; the without-defense, the nudity and the misery of the other. It is also the commandment to take the other upon oneself, not to let him alone; you hear the word of God. If you conceive of the face as the object of a photographer, of course you are dealing with an object like any other object. But if you *encounter* the face, responsibility arises in the strangeness of the other and in his misery. The face offers itself to your compassion and to your obligation.[25]

To understand what Levinas means by face, imagine how Anna sees her friend Barbara Rosenblum as she helps her through the hospital when Barbara is numb from the news of her cancer diagnosis. Anna's responsibility arises in the strangeness that Barbara feels toward herself, and in her misery. Barbara's face is "the exposure to death . . . the without-defense" that offers itself to Anna's compassion and that makes itself her obligation. Crucial to the ethical demand of the face is recognition of the other as always "weaker than you are" (161).[26]

Levinas hears the ethical obligation to the face in mundane injunctions to be nice to other people: "Is not the first word *bonjour*? As simple as *bonjour*. *Bonjour* as benediction and my being available for the other man" (47). But he then radicalizes these courtesies: "the certitude that one must yield to the other the first place in everything, from the *après vous* before an open door right up to the disposition— hardly possible, but holiness demands it—to die for the other" (47; see also 127, among other similar statements). The constant theme of Levinas's writing is this "reversal of the normal order of things" (47). It's normal to seek to preserve our own existence first. To yield to the other the first place in everything, even unto death, is not normal. But in Levinas's ethic, holiness demands no less.

In his interviews Levinas repeatedly quotes Dostoevsky's novel *The Brothers Karamazov*: "Each of us is guilty before everyone and for everything, and I more than all the others" (56; among other references, see especially 112). This sense of guilt underlies the seriousness of the question "Is it righteous to be?" that is the title of Levinas's collected interviews. Explaining this question, Levinas writes that Kafka "describes a culpability without crime, a world in which man never gets to know the accusations charged against him. . . . It is not only the question, 'Is my life righteous?' but rather, 'Is it righteous to be?'" (163).[27]

Levinas's questioning the righteousness of being alive may lead many to share the reaction of François Poirié, a highly informed interviewer, who responds to Levinas: "But it is a crazy demand!" (54) Levinas's philosophy reads to me as an exercise—again in the Stoic sense of a spiritual training—to push this craziness to its human limit. Levinas's practical value lies not at the extremes—we can certainly question whether obligation must be infused with guilt—but in his capacity to underscore the fullest ethical implications of dialogical connection. Levinas himself seems to regard guilt as more heuristic than literal when he writes: "The other engages you in a situation where you are obligated without culpability, but your obligation is not less for all that" (216).

Levinas's question Is it righteous to be? keeps us aware of the innumerable ways that humans usurp each other. From conversational interruptions to inequities of resource consumption to imperialistic wars, humans usurp. The inevitability and the dangers of usurpation are always foremost in Levinas's thinking. Human obligation is to help the other who is weaker than I, in part (at least) because I have already usurped what that other needs. I must offer this help without compounding the original inequity by usurping what is other about that person. "Despite our exchanges, he remains that which I—closed up in myself—am not" (191), Levinas writes, echoing Bakhtin's injunction against the fusion of consciousnesses. Levinas distinguishes himself from Martin Buber because he emphasizes both this enclosure of the self in itself and the asymmetry of the relation of obligation. Levinas describes Buber's I-Thou relation: "we are from the outset in society with each other, but this is a society in which we are equals . . . I am to the other what the other is to me" (213).[28] Instead of Buber's equality, Levinas's imagination of dialogical relations sees "the asymmetry of the I-Thou relation and the radical inequality between the I and the Thou, for every relation is a relation with a being toward whom I have obligations" (213).

Here is why Levinas can be claimed as the fundamental theorist of generosity: his ethical vision of generosity's asymmetry. "I am generous toward the other without this generosity being immediately claimed as reciprocal. . . . I therefore insist upon the signification of this gratuitousness of the *for-the-other* . . . " (213, emphasis in the original).

Bakhtin seems closer to Buber than to Levinas. Bakhtin emphasizes the self's "nonself-sufficiency, the impossibility of the existence of a single consciousness. I am conscious of myself and become myself only while revealing myself for another, through another, and with the help of another."[29] Levinas would, I think, read Bakhtin's "with the help of" as undercutting "this *gratuitousness*" (quoted above; emphasis added) of being for-the-other. If I am receiving the other's help, then I am less than fully for-the-other. The quality of gratuitousness is the radical demand in Levinas's ethics; it becomes the benchmark of what is truly moral.[30]

Why does Levinas need to make his demand so crazy in its insistence on nonreciprocity? Although Bakhtin had some measure of Stalin's terror inflicted on him, Levinas seems more self-conscious of writing after Auschwitz. One implication of writing in this constant shadow is Levinas's understanding of the other person, the face, as "being exposed to the point of death" (145). A complementary issue is the problem of affirmation. Levinas writes with a grief that can never be resolved: "One wonders afterward [after the *shoah*, the Holocaust] if it is still possible to uphold something" (197). Levinas seems to believe that anything worth upholding must be radical in its response to a world in which so many people, and people so specifically chosen, were abandoned to their death. Those of us who live after are not culpable, yet we share the human nature, the "genus" as Levinas calls it, of those who were guilty. The righteousness of our own being is always in question.

The generous self for Levinas is "the hostage of the other," and again, a hostage without reciprocity (132–33; see also 204). The hostage is the "first one called" to care for the other, and to be called is to be "the chosen one" (153). This quality of being hostage, being chosen, is the foundation of both the individual and of society.[31] But a society of the chosen would encounter a problem that Levinas repeatedly acknowledges: "We are not a pair, alone in the world, but at least three" (193). This third person is "also my neighbor" (115), and with his presence, "the other's singularity is placed in question. I must look him [the third] in the face as well" (133).

The requirement to look the third person in the face gives rise to the demand of justice. On Levinas's account, justice is necessary but impossible. No one can "compare the incomparable" (133; see also 166), and so "justice constantly has a bad conscience" (194). At the extreme, justice is violence (167). Yet charity, Levinas repeats, requires justice (205) and is fulfilled in justice (194). The last chapter of this book returns to the problem of how justice can retain its foundation in the obligation to respect the incomparability of the face.

Throughout his life Levinas, whose first written language was Hebrew, wrote both philosophy and religion—Talmudic studies and topical essays on Judaism. He attempted to keep these streams separate, even having two publishers. In my favorite critical essay on Levinas, philosopher Hilary Putnam questions both the success and the value of this separation: "It is part of Levinas's strategy to regularly transfer predicates to the other [person] that traditional theology ascribes to God."[32] As theology depicts humans perpetually obligated to God, Levinas transfers this obligation to other persons. Holiness is found in the face and obligations to it.

Putnam underscores the difference between Levinas's relation to others and the Stoic primacy of rendering yourself beyond disturbance.

For Levinas, the experience of the other as, in effect, a violator of his mind, as one who breaks his phenomenology, goes with what I called the "fundamental obligation" to make oneself available to the other, and with the experience of what Levinas calls "the Glory of the Infinite." (42)

Levinas might sound, as another interviewer says, simply utopian.[33] Yet as the stories in chapters 4 and 5 will show, practical decisions of care can require making yourself available to the other who may be "a violator." The guest may break out of the containment strategies that seem reasonable and call into question the limits of obligation. Levinas is the indispensable theorist of the limits of dialogue and generosity. He requires us to confront his crazy demand that there are no limits to obligation.

Too Much Discipline?

Before the Dialogical Stoic is put to work reflecting on stories of illness and care, two caveats and one response to an anticipated objection can be added. First, I neither minimize nor emphasize the differences between Marcus's Stoic ethics and dialogical ethics, or between Bakhtin and Levinas. Lest I set up Levinas as the patron saint of responsibility for others and relegate Marcus's value to moments of solitude, let me quote Marcus's reminder to himself: "To move from one unselfish action to another with God in mind. Only there, delight and stillness" (vi.7). Levinas could find no better epigraph.

Second, lest the emphasis on dialogue afford undue privilege to language, I note that Bakhtin writes: "Dialogic relationships . . . are extralinguistic," and below that, partially explaining it, "judgments must be embodied."[34] Sam Crane's story of washing Aidan exemplifies such extralinguistic dialogue. Even when care and consolation are expressed in language, generosity is extralinguistic.

Third and perhaps most open to dialogical contestation: What about the objection that the Dialogical Stoic is too much a creature of self-imposed disciplines and obligations, two unfashionable words that make people nervous? Don't ill people have enough trouble without having to become Stoics, and don't those who care for them have enough demands without being told to worry about whether they are fulfilling conditions of dialogue? To these humane concerns I can only answer: Here we are; how do we act like humans? Part of what I love about "The Tunnel" is how its characters find themselves called to dialogue by a situation they have not chosen. But there they are, in the tunnel. When we go through such tunnels together, dialogue is not a choice, in the sense of an optional extra. Dialogue is a demand (another unpopular word) that attends being a human among humans. It's not "one more thing" but the *one* thing. Stop complaining, I imagine Marcus saying. Will you behave like a human being, and if not, what are you behaving like, and do you really want *that*?

Stoicism and dialogical thinking are disciplines insofar as they call for going beyond abstract knowledge and asking yourself to change your ideas and your habits (because for the Stoics, you can change your ideas only by changing your habits). *Doing* is what counts, and knowing what counts as worth doing depends on being a person who has become shaped through discipline. Stoic and dialogical training values acting in ways that most people consider counterintuitive. It's intuitive to react to representations; Marcus provides a practice for training ourselves to interrupt those reactions and decide which judgments we choose to hold on to and which we will consider not conducive to becoming who we want to be. This Stoic discipline of assent is not an extra demand on ill people; it's a practical necessity. The alternative is to remain perpetually vulnerable to being plunged back into the shock that Barbara Rosenblum experiences on hearing her diagnosis. Universal Stoicism asks whether you want to go on being shocked by every new representation of illness; if not, what are you willing to do to train yourself to act otherwise?

It is also intuitive to understand obligations as reciprocal. Making yourself hostage to the need of the other is counterintuitive. It's counterintuitive to drop your carefully acquired tone, the tone that gives you status in some hierarchy, and speak *with* another person. Thinking of yourself without internal sovereignty, without clear boundary between your self and the other, is counterintuitive. But the stories in the chapters that follow show people making the leap into such counterintuitive understanding and action, and finding consolation in having made that leap.

A gentler closing is provided by Marcus's quotation (vi.24) from the philosopher Heraclitus: "Even a soul submerged in sleep is hard at work, and helps to make something of the world."[35] From this perspective, there is no discipline at all; no demands and no comparison of attainments, since each does its part. Awake or asleep, each soul is hard at its work. Marcus trains himself not to question who plays what role; think instead how soon all will return to smoke. But until then, his assignment is to help make something of the world. That is all the Dialogical Stoic asks.

CHAPTER THREE

The Generosity of the Ill

W HEN people get sick, they want to get well. Getting well may be all some ever want. But some whose world is taken apart by sickness want the world they put back together to be different. They feel blessed to be alive and they want to return this generosity. When Lance Armstrong, in the story told in

> *Whatever impedes*
> *action can advance it.*
> *Your mind can turn*
> *whatever stands in the*
> *way into the way.*
> MARCUS AURELIUS
>
> ✿

chapter 1, realizes that cancer is not his isolated problem and feels "increased companionship with [his] fellow patients," he sees his life as having different stakes. He still wants to win bike races, but he wants more. Cancer is more than errant cells inside his body requiring treatment. Cancer becomes a human problem that he is called to respond to. His illness becomes an occasion for generosity.

Armstrong's oncologist asks him to reflect on the "obligations of the cured." Whether or not either of them realizes it, these words paraphrase what Albert Schweitzer wrote decades earlier. Schweitzer—the great theologian, Bach scholar, and organist—attended medical school in midlife and became most famous as a medical missionary in Africa, winning the Nobel Peace Prize in 1952. Although Schweitzer was German, his first medical mission was sponsored by the Paris Missionary Society and founded in a French colony. When World War I began, he was respectfully but firmly interned for the duration. The deprivations of this experience left him seriously ill, requiring multiple surgeries and several years' recuperation. Schweitzer describes how his illness affected his sense of obligation to others:

The Fellowship of those who bear the Mark of Pain. Who are the members of this Fellowship? Those who have learnt by experience what physical pain and bodily anguish mean, belong together all the world over; they are united by a secret bond. One and all they know the horrors of suffering to which man can be exposed, and one and all they know the longing to be free from pain. He who has been delivered from pain must not think he is now free again, and at liberty to take life up just as it was before, entirely forgetful of the past. He is now a "man whose eyes are open" with regard to pain and anguish, and he must help to overcome those two enemies (so far as human power can control them) and to bring to others the deliverance which he has himself enjoyed.[1]

Schweitzer imagines illness in the Stoic manner that this chapter's epigraph expresses: he transforms the illness that was the obstacle *in* his way into the calling that sets him *on* the way. In the following passage, Schweitzer separates what is inner from what is exterior, finds freedom in the inner, and seeks to be beyond susceptibility to disturbance caused by the external:

True resignation consists in this: that man, feeling his subordination to the course of world events, makes his way toward inward freedom from the fate that shapes his external existence. Inward freedom gives him the strength to triumph over the difficulties of everyday life and to become a deeper and more inward person, calm and peaceful. Resignation, therefore, is the spiritual and ethical affirmation of one's own existence. Only he who has gone through a trial of resignation is capable of accepting the world.[2]

Schweitzer must have gone through one "trial of resignation" when he made his decision to give up an acclaimed academic and musical career. He went to Africa to carve a hospital out of the jungle and practice medicine under the most exacting and hazardous conditions. About these conditions he is generally stoic in the colloquial sense of not complaining, but he provides occasional descriptions of life in his medical mission:

Our own health [Schweitzer's and his wife's] is not first-class, though it is not really bad; tropical anemia has, indeed, already set in. It shows itself in the way the slightest exertion tires one; I am quite exhausted [the passage describes events in 1915, when Schweitzer was 40], for example, after coming up the hill to my house, a matter of four minutes' walk. We also perceive in ourselves a symptom that accompanies it, an excessive nervousness, and besides these two things we find that our teeth are in a bad condition. My wife and I put temporary fillings into each other's teeth, and in this way I gave her some relief, but no one can do for me what is really necessary. . . . What stories could be told of toothache in the forest! [3]

"People who love what they do wear themselves down doing it" (v.1), wrote Marcus Aurelius. Fortunately Schweitzer's health improved, and he was active until he died at 90.

Schweitzer's sense of obligation may begin in an eternal Stoicism, but he does not remain within the "internal dialogicality" that Bakhtin considers characteristic of the Stoics. What Bakhtin calls the Stoic "discovery of the inner man" is not an end in itself for Schweitzer, but only instigates and orients his responsibility to others.[4] Schweitzer decides to abandon academia and Europe in order to define himself in a relation of care to others: "I must establish a relationship with my life in this world, insofar as it is within my reach, one that is not only passive but active."[5] The person who takes this active role "is united with the lives that surround him; *he experiences the destinies of others as his own*" (233, emphases added).

This statement is echoed by Levinas, speaking in an interview in 1983: "I don't very much like the word *love,* which is worn out and debased. Let us speak instead of the *taking upon oneself the fate of the other.*"[6] When Schweitzer goes to Africa as a medical missionary, he takes upon himself the fate of the other. Schweitzer writes that after his illness, his life "no longer belongs to himself alone."[7] This conjunction of Schweitzer and Levinas exemplifies what Hilary Putnam calls Levinas's moral perfectionism.[8] Moral perfectionists do not believe that only perfection is acceptable, or even that it is attainable. They do believe that humans need to sustain a vision of as much perfection as is imaginable, if we are to become fully human. Putnam writes:

Moral perfectionists believe that the ancient questions—"Am I living as I am supposed to live?" "Is my life something more than vanity, or worse, mere conformity?" "Am I making the best effort I can to reach . . . my unattained but attainable self?"—make all the difference in the world. . . . Such a philosopher is a "perfectionist" because s/he always describes the commitment we ought to have in ways that seem impossibly demanding; but such a philosopher is also a realist, because s/he realizes that it is only by keeping an "impossible" demand in view that one can strive for one's "unattained but attainable self." (36)

This book is populated by moral perfectionists, from Fabiola to those whose stories are told in this chapter and the following ones. The phrase "moral perfectionism" sounds heavy to contemporary ears; it seems to impose a burden, like Schweitzer's fellowship of those who bear the mark of pain. Such phrases do assert a radical ideal of responsibility, and the line between inspiring and burdening may necessarily be a fine one.

Moral perfectionism claims the significance of an ideal, but it *does not judge* any individual's actual attainments. Schweitzer and Levinas do not judge; one exception is Levinas's moral imperative to judge responsibility for the Holocaust. Their *realism*, as Putnam calls it, is to recognize the need to keep "impossible" demands clearly in view. They seek to illuminate moral possibility, not to impose moral burdens. They bear witness to the shift reported by many people who are committed to lives of service: there is no burden; instead, a peaceful sense of living life in the only way that feels right. That sense of rightness lightens life.

Schweitzer's fellowship of those who bear the mark of pain describes those whom Levinas calls *chosen:* "he is chosen because he was the first to hear the call"[9]—the call, that is, of the other's suffering and need. Hearing this call and recognizing oneself as chosen instigates the "crisis of resignation" that Schweitzer evokes. To hear the call is to resign yourself to obligation, because you realize that obligation is the only way to save your life. Levinas explains:

I believe that if one looks closely at the prophetic [biblical] texts, one sees that they always describe the other as weaker than you are. I am always obligated to him. In *The Brothers Karamazov,* Dostoevsky says that we are all responsible for everything, before everyone, and I more than all the others. I am always responsible, each I is noninterchangeable. Nothing else can do what I do in my place. The knot of singularity is responsibility. (161)

For Levinas, all humans are chosen, though clearly some hear the call sooner than others.

All are chosen because our human sense of extensive obligation— obligation to others whom we do not know—makes our condition unique. Levinas expresses what it is to be human in a rhetorical question that describes who the human always already is:

Or is the I posited straightaway for-the-other, straightaway in obligation and straightaway as the only one who is ready to respond and to bear responsibility, like one who is the first to have hearkened to the call and the last, perhaps, to have listened to it? (117–18)

This chapter describes people whose own experience of illness leads them "to respond and to bear responsibility." Outward response, with responsibility for others, has a necessary complement in inner dialogue. Reynolds Price exemplifies those whose response to illness—while no less a "hearkening to the call"—hearkens inward, in order to turn outward. He shows others who are in pain what inner resources they can discover for themselves.

Price, an eminent playwright, novelist, and poet, had cancer within his spinal cord. The horrific treatment includes surgery and radiation that leave him in stable remission but in chronic pain and paralyzed from midchest down. His memoir of illness and disability evokes the ill person's abandonment within him- or herself—the times alone that I described in chapter 2. "I need steady coaching," Price writes; "I'm never home free."[10] Like Marcus, he coaches in a second-person voice that addresses himself as much as it speaks to others who suffer:

You're in your present calamity alone, far as this life goes. If you want a way out, then dig it yourself. . . . Nobody—least of all a doctor—can rescue you now, not from the depths of your own mind, not once they've stitched your gaping wound. (182)

In the Stoic manner, Price finds healing by changing his own beliefs about his situation. You begin digging yourself out, he advises, first by allowing yourself to grieve "for a decent limited time over whatever parts of your old self you know you'll miss."

Then find your way to be somebody else, the next viable you—a stripped-down whole other clear-eyed person, realistic as a sawed-off shotgun and thankful for air, not to speak of the human kindness you'll meet if you get normal luck. (183)

I imagine Marcus especially liking the parts about remaking the self as stripped-down, clear-eyed, and realistic, all good Stoic ideals. And Marcus, ever the warrior, would be comfortable with the sawed-off shotgun metaphor.

"Who'll you be tomorrow?" (182) is the question that Price proposes can save the life of someone who has suffered the sort of devastating illness he has.[11] Some of the selves you can be tomorrow are better than some other selves you might be. At minimum, it's better to be a new self who has grieved and buried those parts of the old that are gone. But regardless of the content of the self, by centering the experience of illness on the question—Who will you be? (and who is it good, useful to others, and true to yourself, to be)—Price reclaims his own moral identity.

Price's question—"Who'll you be tomorrow?"—animates all the illness stories discussed below. Others place less faith in their ability to answer this question within themselves and seek their answers through relationships.[12] Illness becomes an occasion for generosity in many ways. Price's generosity lies in offering his uncompromising self-reflection and unsurpassed prose style. This chapter considers efforts to achieve more generous *representations* of the ill and disabled, generosity in expanding the scope of moral *participation* for the ill and disabled, and finally *"health ecology,"* which questions the boundaries of who, or what, is sick and needs healing.

ABSENCE AND REPRESENTATION

Images of illness and disability are generated as part of the complex of representations that any society creates and perpetuates. Individuals are then defined in the terms that these images propose. To understand the stakes that any group has in how it is represented, I begin with a bizarre historical scene, recalled in the writing of Henry Louis Gates, a scholar of African-American studies.[13]

In 1772 eighteen of Boston's most prominent citizens, including both the governor of the colony and John Hancock, whose signature would be the most famous calligraphy on the Declaration of Independence that would end colonial status, met to examine an eighteen-year-old slave woman, Phillis Wheatley. They sought to determine if she was the author of a book of poems that her master, John Wheatley, claimed she had written. Publishers were refusing the poems because the wisdom of the day maintained that an African could not be literate. Wheatley's authorship, therefore, must be a hoax. For the Enlightenment, writing was a privileged sign of reason, and reason was the criterion of full humanity. Africans, so it was believed, lacked sufficient reason to be capable of writing. Thus the political stakes riding on Phillis Wheatley's authorship were high. If she was judged to be the author, then her writing constituted proof that Africans were capable of writing and thus of reason—and acknowledgment of that capability precipitated a strong argument against slavery.

Gates notes that when this panel of distinguished citizens did attest the authenticity of Wheatley's authorship, and the poems were published on the strength of their judgment, "scores of reviews of Wheatley's book argued that the publication of her poems meant that the African was indeed a human being and should not be enslaved" (593). Phillis Wheatley was freed soon after her poems were published, and we can regret that a similar panel of enlightened citizens could not have adjudicated the end of slavery in the United States so peacefully.

Gates concludes his discussion of Phillis Wheatley: "The very face of race was contingent upon the recording of the black voice. Voice presupposed a face" (595). Like Levinas, Gates means more by face than the arrangement of eyes, nose, and mouth. Phillis Wheatley's face includes her vulnerability as a woman and a slave, her weakness in Dostoevsky's sense that the other is always weaker. Her face includes the silence that is imposed on her by how Africans are represented in eighteenth-century America. Recognizing the authenticity of Phillis Wheatley's authorship involved seeing her as a fellow human, fully capable of all human joy, pain, reflection, and insight; and perhaps most of all, capable of suffering injustice. Recognition of that human face is necessary to overcome what Gates calls "blackness as a *sign of absence*" (596, emphases added), and in that idea—some groups are represented by a sign that renders them absent—issues of race converge with illness and disability.

The trial of Phillis Wheatley, sounding so distant at first, raises questions and issues that are contemporary for people who are ill or disabled. These conditions render people liable to being treated as if some part of their self has become absent to others' recognition. Illness and disability, like race, are too often signs of absence. Thus it had to be discovered that medical patients ought to give explicit consent to procedures performed on their bodies.[14] *Representation* is the problem of converting absence into presence and restoring persons to moral recognition. To date, the disability rights movement has done the most to disentangle issues of representation and misrepresentation.[15]

Michael Bérubé is a professor of literature for whom disability instigates a need to reflect on the moral and practical implications of representation. Bérubé tells stories about his son, Jamie, who was born in 1991 with Down syndrome. Bérubé writes: "Individual humans like James are compelling us daily to determine what *kind* of 'individuality' we will value, on what terms, and why."[16] Jamie's birth lands him at what his father calls a "busy intersection" of institutions and knowl-edges, all bidding to define Jamie's individuality and how he will be valued. Among these institutions and knowledges, Bérubé includes "statutes, allocations, genetics, reproduction" (xix), each with its own interest in how Jamie is represented. This competition generates Bérubé's task: to represent his son generously, lest others do so with-out generosity.

Bérubé uses the language of obligation to explain how he became chosen, in Levinas's sense, by Jamie's vulnerability to others' repre-sentations of him:

> Perhaps those of us who can understand this intersection have an obligation to "represent" the children who can't. . . . As those children grow, perhaps we need to foster their abilities to represent themselves—and to listen to them as they do. I strongly suspect we do have those obligations. I am not entirely sure what they might entail. But it is part of my purpose, in writing this book, to represent Jamie as best I can—just as it is part of my purpose, in representing Jamie, to ask ques-tions about our obligations to each other, individually and socially, and about our capacity to imagine other people. . . . I know how crucial it is that we collectively cultivate our capacities to imagine our obligations to each other. (xix)

Bérubé required Jamie's presence in his life in order to imagine his ob-ligations to someone like Jamie. For the rest of us to imagine our obli-gations to Jamie and people like him, we require stories that make Jamie's life narratable.

Narratable is a word Bérubé uses to remind us that social conven-tions determine what's worth telling a story about: not everything that everybody does is seen by others as worthy of a story.[17] Stories do not merely narrate events. They convey on action and actor—either one or both—the socially accredited status of being worth notice. To ren-der narratable is to claim relevance for an action, and for the life of which that action is part. Storytelling continually redraws the bound-aries of a community's recognitions; it renders present what would otherwise be absent. As recognitions change, so do obligations. An ob-ligation presupposes a face, and a face presupposes a story.

Jamie's disability was a surprise. Bérubé writes of his amused con-cern while his wife was pregnant with Jamie, their second child, that they might fall into a typical pattern of parents who can't muster the same level of enthusiasm about this child's developmental milestones.

Parents' scrapbooks of their second child are often far thinner than those of the firstborn. "But everything was changed, changed utterly," he writes. "Jamie's milestones were every bit as amazing and . . . as narratable as were Nick's [Jamie's older brother]" (127).

If Jamie's milestones are narratable, it's because of the representations that his father and others—like Sam Crane—have created. Had Jamie been born not so many years earlier, or at the same time but in a different place, to different parents who were given different advice, he would have been institutionalized with no expectation that he would develop or accomplish milestones. We hear the echo of Phillis Wheatley, who was assumed by most of the people of her time to be incapable of literacy. Today as in 1772, the political stakes on narratability are high, including allocation of educational and other resources.

"My task," Bérubé writes, "ethically and aesthetically, is to represent James to you with all the fidelity that mere language can afford, the better to enable you to imagine him—and to imagine what he might think of your ability to imagine him" (264). The task of representation is both ethical and aesthetic. What we think counts for ethical consideration depends on how it is represented, and representations necessarily have an aesthetic dimension. Bérubé's last clause is equally important, because until we can imagine other people evaluating how we imagine them—until we credit the other person with an imagination of us—those people are not seen as faces to which we have obligations. In "The Tunnel," told in chapter 1, the young physician can imagine his patient imagining the tunnel and what happens there, but he does not seem to imagine his patient imagining *him* and how he acts.

How imaginations interact in the clinic is expressed by Anatole Broyard, distinguished literary critic and author, who died of prostate cancer. Broyard was certainly capable of representing himself, but he realized that once he became a patient, part of him was rendered absent, at least to his physicians. Speaking to physicians about his experiences, Broyard reminds them that their patients are evaluating how they, as physicians, imagine them: "While he invariably feels superior to me because he is the doctor and I am the patient, I'd like him to know that I feel superior to him, too, that he is my patient also and I have my diagnosis of him."[18] Broyard realizes that until physicians see their patients as people who are diagnosing them, illness will remain a sign of absence. "Without some such recognition," Broyard pleads, "I am nothing but my illness" (45). In Broyard's "nothing but" I hear the echo of Phillis Wheatley and the lifelong problem of Jamie Bérubé.

The stakes in representation involve specific dangers to people whose lives can depend on how they are represented.[19] Phillis Wheatley was in danger in Boston in 1772, even with a "master" who apparently valued her as a person. Danger is the background of Jamie Bérubé's life. This danger is expressed in a book Michael Bérubé introduces, written by Jason Kingsley and Mitchell Levitz, two teen-agers (at the time of writing) with Down's.[20] The book records conversations between Jason and Mitchell, and sometimes with other members of their families, transcribed and edited by their mothers for length but not for expression.

Jason Kingsley expresses the danger with which a person who has Down syndrome lives when he speaks of "the obstetrician [who] said that I cannot learn" and advised sending Jason to an institution.[21] Jason details the many things he has done and learned, his musical accomplishments, his friendships, and his appreciations. "So I want the obstetrician will never say that to any parent to have a baby with a disability any more. If you send a baby with a disability to an institution, the baby will miss all the opportunities to grow and to learn" (28). This passage elicits what Levinas calls "fearing for the other."[22] Moral obligation begins in that fear. Moral indifference is never having encountered a representation that elicits that fear.

Moral Participation

Kingsley and Levitz's title, *Count Us In*, expresses the problem that people who are ill or disabled have staying *in* networks of participation, and participating on terms that are meaningful to themselves and are recognized as meaningful by others. Essayist Nancy Mairs, whose body is impaired by advanced multiple sclerosis, expresses the stakes riding on participation. "I can't become a 'hopeless cripple,'" she writes, "without risking moral paralysis."[23] Disability poses a threat to Mairs's moral participation in the world; participation is the means and medium of being moral. She presupposes what Marcus Aurelius denies: for her to be moral, others must recognize her moral capacity.

The medium and means of Mairs's participation is her body, which is "in trouble" (42). At the time Mairs writes, she is capable of thinking, speaking, and writing, and she retains the unimpaired use of one arm. This body-in-trouble causes her to be fearful: "I have visions of enduring life at the hands of strangers: refused food or drink, shoved roughly into bed, allowed to slip from my wheelchair and abandoned in a puddle of my own urine" (56).[24] But Mairs's fears go beyond the risks of institutionalization. Her body is the vehicle for dialogical engagement with others. As this body becomes more troubled, she risks the "moral paralysis" that is her deeper fear.

If I don't want to be reduced to a constellation of problems, I must imagine my body as something other than problematic: a vehicle for enmeshing the life I have been given into the lives of others. Easy enough to say. But to do? Who will have me? And on what terms? (56)

Mairs is clear that the nondisabled world (her term of choice) cares little about her participation, moral or otherwise. People take a "dismissive attitude" toward others who, in their wheelchairs, "live at the height of your waist" (62).[25] Mairs's disability places her under a sign of moral absence:

Beyond cheerfulness and patience, people don't generally expect much of a cripple's character. And certainly they presume that care, which I have placed at the heart of moral experience, flows in one direction, "downward": as from adult to child, so from well to ill, from whole to maimed. (62)

Mairs places care at "the heart of moral experience," and she equates "downward" care with failure to recognize the person being cared for as a moral presence, not a body in which the human is currently absent. When the moral presence is judged to be absent, the body can be refused food and drink, shoved roughly into bed, and allowed to sit in its own urine. Such a body becomes "it"—no longer *you*, no longer a face.

The asymmetry that is inherent in most medical care means that care cannot be mutual in a material sense, but each party to a relation of care can imagine the other as having something to contribute to the needs of the world. Mairs finds a community embodying that recognition among Catholic Workers: "a community that . . . assum[es] that the moral core of being in the world lies in the care of others, in *doing* good rather than *being* good" (61). But this emphasis on doing, while it solves the problem of how to judge what "being good" means, creates another problem. Mairs's participation in this community stands to be blocked by her body in trouble: "How can a woman identify herself as a Catholic Worker," she wonders, "if she can't even cut up carrots for the soup or ladle it out for the hungry people queued up outside the kitchen door? Physical incapacity certainly appears to rob such a woman of moral efficacy" (62).

Mairs recognizes that for her to be "excused" from *doing* good would deny her moral participation, even when that excuse is "on the most generous of grounds: that she suffers enough already" (62). To excuse her is to dismiss her. To "enable or require me to withdraw from moral life altogether" (63) is a violence, however benevolent the intent. Mairs's "enable or require" usage is crucial to her argument. To *enable* her to withdraw is as morally injurious to her as *requiring* her to withdraw. She needs moral participation in order to exist as fully human, however troubled in body.

Mairs's solution lies in the different capacities arising from each person's singularity. She can't make soup, but she can write. "What I can still *do*—so far—is write books. Catholic Workers being extraordinarily tolerant of multiplicity, on the theory that it takes all kinds of parts to form a body, this activity will probably be counted good enough" (63). A happy ending: those who cannot serve soup can find moral participation in writing, and those who are better at serving soup than at spinning personal experience into moral philosophy can do so, with no denigration of anyone's participation.

Yet how happy is this ending? In Mairs's assessment of what is "counted good enough," Levinas might hear an intimation of "that which I am for you, you are for me," a reciprocity that deteriorates into an economic relation of "adding-up." [26] Levinas's interviewer characterizes this relation as an "exchange of wares" (150). Levinas's doubts about basing mutual responsibility on reciprocity—no matter how tolerant of multiplicity—are practical problems for Mairs. Her qualification of what she can do "so far" is an ominous note. What happens to her moral participation when, for reasons physical or intellectual, she loses writing as her distinct form of participation? Then she will need a world that defines moral participation without any reciprocity; a world where downward care—Levinas's insistence that the other is always weaker—retains a vision of the human face, and being a face is enough to create an obligation of care.

In one of Mairs's earlier books she suggests caring relationships that are closer to Levinas's ideal of nonreciprocity.[27] She reinterprets reciprocity as a meeting of complementary "abundances." Everyone has abundances. What many people—the homeless, the sick, the disabled—have an abundance of is need, but that fits the system of reciprocity. Mairs's Levinasian premise is that humans have a need to give; the other person's lack thus fills that need. "Of course," she writes with a Stoic wit, "an abundance may not take the form you much like" (163). She recalls an unpleasant encounter she had with a homeless person who might have been a panhandler—in some cases a difference of representation. She had little taste for filling his abundance of need, which was probably for alcohol; nor did he like how she filled it, with an offer of health food she had just purchased. Her point, which I think Levinas would appreciate, is that liking it has nothing to do with moral participation.

Participation, Mairs concludes, depends on generosity. "My infinitely harder task," she writes, "is to conceptualize not merely a habitable body but a habitable world: a world that wants me in it."[28] The medical world is not yet habitable; patients are too often treated as if they are not wanted. One testimony to such treatment comes from Evan Handler, describing his treatment for leukemia. Handler experienced the repeated denial of his need to participate in his own healing. Finally he meets a physician who, to Handler's surprise, "invited me to participate with him in his investigation. Not merely to endure it. Not make myself scarce while he had a go at my body. But rather, to allow him to try to help me by joining him in the attempt."[29] Generous physicians may not *do* anything very differently from how their colleagues do it. But they do it generously, and the difference is palpable, literally so, on this occasion.

Handler wants a physician who will not regard his disease as a sign of absence that spreads over his whole being. He tells a psychiatrist that he wants a physician "who will understand all the other things I'm doing." The response is a pithy statement of medicine's demoralization: "You won't find it there," the psychiatrist says of the cancer treatment center. "You find a way to use them as best you can. You will know if you've found a doctor you can use. You don't have to tell them about yourself. They can't handle it" (100). As Handler's story of treatment unfolds, he seems to be better off the more he follows this advice.

Ultimately he creates his participation by writing his book. Writing is Handler's remoralization, and the pity is that it had to occur after and outside of his medical treatment. Handler had to suffer through being demoralized before he could remoralize himself. The physicians who treated him—his nurses varied—were not part of a remoralization that might have affected their lives.

Generosity in how ill and disabled people are represented opens possibilities for their participation, and their participation expands the scope of society's generosity. The next level of generosity redefines health, illness, and death. Bérubé and Mairs anticipate this redefinition, but other writers make it explicit.

HEALTH ECOLOGY

Tim Brookes coins the term *health ecology* to imagine a new form of medicine that would reflect what he has learned, first from living with asthma himself, and then from "going global" in understanding asthma as more than his personal problem.[30] As a patient he wants the benefits of mainstream medicine, but he is demoralized when his doctors define him in terms of his compliance with standardized directives. Brookes wants to be more than compliant: "If I've become a success story," he writes, "it's because I have become engaged in the process of healing" (277). Like Mairs and Handler, Brookes wants participation.

Many people living with illness differentiate healing from cure, the key distinction being that healing involves the ill or disabled person's participation. Health ecology poses the question, participation in what? What is the network of connections that the ill person participates in? How does disease originate in a network of connections, and how must healing involve recognizing the person's place in this network? *Ecology*, as it pertains to health, is another word for the moral necessity of dialogue, in Bakhtin's sense of people acting with the awareness that their lives are lived wholly on the boundary with others. Health ecology expands those others to include the earth itself.

Illness, Brookes comes to understand, "presents an opportunity to learn about ourselves and the world we inhabit and create" (277). The conjunctions in this statement are dialogical. Brookes first links self to world, and then proposes that as we inhabit our world, we constantly recreate it. Another definition of ecology is taking responsibility for how we recreate; specifically, what values guide our work of recreating life. Health ecology requires being awake to the moral risk and the possibility inherent in how we recreate not only our own lives but life itself. Brookes imagines that medical schools might someday include a new discipline of health ecology.

Health ecology begins with what Paul Komesaroff calls the "continuous flow of ethical decisions" that make up medical practice.[31] "It would study the way patients listen to doctors, and vice versa," Brookes says, "and the way patients speak to doctors, and vice versa."[32] Brookes is aware that a huge literature exists on doctor-patient communication, but in his departments of Health Ecology, this warhorse topic would be studied differently, because the auspice would be moral, and the communication would flow both ways.

Brookes begins with his own asthma attacks and goes into operating rooms to watch lung surgery and to low-income neighborhoods to observe public health units. "After all," he writes at the end of this journey, "Health Ecology assumes that neither the asthmatic nor his environment can ever suffer alone" (284). Brookes's morality is fully dialogical:

If, as individuals or as a society, or as a species we don't understand ourselves, some of us will always be unhealthy, and all of us will suffer, even (though less obviously) those who prosper and profit from others' disease. Healing is a collective activity, not a commodity—a verb, not a noun. When one person falls ill or stays healthy, the entire universe is involved. (284)[33]

Health ecology shifts the responsibility inherent in Schweitzer's fellowship of those who bear the mark of pain from the ill to everyone. Those who happen to be ill now are Levinas's chosen: they are the first to realize that their suffering is ultimately everyone's suffering. Ill people may hear the call first, but the call is for everyone. No one can be healthy until each fears for the other and feels obligated to the other. That obligation is health.

Terry Tempest Williams and Vanessa Kramer expand Brookes's insight that when one person falls ill, the entire universe is involved. Each understands that pathology inside the body results from, and mirrors, relationships among bodies, earth, and history. Some of these relationships are distorted, and others are the way life is. Our contemporary problem is confusion over what is unnatural and what's

natural. Williams and Kramer understand health as *truth* about how
history is known and how the world is recreated. They show why
health-as-truth has to be generous; otherwise it's untrue.

The ecological consciousness of illness is clear in the title of Terry
Tempest Williams's *Refuge: An Unnatural History of Family and
Place*. The place in the title, her place, is the Great Salt Lake region of
Utah, which Williams studies in her work as a naturalist. Her family
are descendents of the original Mormon settlers. What the title calls
unnatural is the death rate from cancer. "At thirty-four," Williams
writes, "I became the matriarch of my family."[34] The older women
have all died from breast cancer. Williams's story is how this cancer is
entwined with the history of the land. Like the other stories in this
chapter, it is about fear, representation, and participation.

Williams's fear of cancer pervades her life. She dreams of being
told: "You have cancer in your blood and you have nine months to heal
yourself" (3), a symbolic length of time that reappears in her story.
Cancer is in her blood—the blood she shares with the other women in
her family—whether or not she ever has what medicine calls cancer.
In Williams's dream the phantom doctor merely delivers the message;
the responsibility to heal falls on her. Williams makes writing the medium of this self-healing: "Perhaps, I am telling this story in an attempt to heal myself, to confront what I do not know, to create a path
for myself with the idea that 'memory is the only way home'" (4).

The home Williams grew up in is a loving place, but it harbors silence about a misrecognition. Given the stakes, this misrecognition assumes the force of a lie. Late in the book, after Williams has evoked the
deaths of many of her family members from cancer and, in her book's
parallel theme, the ecological degradation of the Great Salt Lake region, she describes another dream. She tells her father about her re-
curring dream of a bright light in the sky. He replies that the dream is
a memory of the family watching an atomic bomb explode. "We pulled
[the car] over," he tells her, "and suddenly, rising from the desert floor,
we saw it, clearly, this golden-stemmed cloud, the mushroom. The sky
seemed to vibrate with an eerie pink glow. Within a few minutes, a
light ash was raining on the car." She stares at him. "I thought you
knew that," he says; "it was a common occurrence in the fifties" (283).

It was at this moment that I realized the deceit I had been living under. Children
growing up in the American Southwest, drinking contaminated milk from con-

taminated cows, even from the contaminated breasts of their mothers, my
mother—members, years later, of the Clan of One-Breasted Women. (283)

Once Williams knows this truth, she seeks a form of participation
that is both moral witness and protest. *Refuge* ends when she and
other women are arrested for picketing a nuclear test site in Nevada.
Williams's participation sets her against the Mormon tradition of adherence to authority, but the protest is essential to her healing. In it
she self-consciously risks her body in order to reclaim herself from the
risks that continue to be imposed on the bodies of her family without
their knowledge or consent. The women's cancer derives from an insult
to the earth, and so healing must begin with the earth.

Williams describes this conjunction of the body of the earth and the
physical body, particularly the maternal body, as the motivation to
protest:

The women couldn't bear it any longer. They were mothers. They had suffered
labor pains but always under the promise of birth. The red hot pains beneath the
desert promised death only, as each bomb became a stillborn. A contract had been
made and broken between human beings and the land. A new contract was being
drawn by the women, who understood the fate of the earth as their own. (288)

This need for a new and generous contract is developed in Vanessa
Kramer's remarkable essay about medical demoralization and the ecological awareness necessary to remoralize both medicine and the spirit
of how humans live as parts of the earth. Kramer writes between re-
currences of breast cancer. She shares Williams's family history:
"When I was a small child, I lived with my parents in my grandmother's house in England. Of the six women in the house at that time,
four of us have developed cancer over the years. Now only one of the
four survives." [35]

In the first part of her essay, Kramer tells a story about her aunt's
treatment for ovarian cancer. In the second part she makes an ecological case against toxic treatments, especially radiation, as cancer therapy. Both parts are unified by problems of death. Problems, that is, not
of death itself, but of the silence about death that pervades cancer
centers: "that loud silence that makes most cancer wards so bizarre, if
you are paying attention" (1). Kramer's thesis (in my terms) is that
medicine demoralizes because it has no place for death, and thus no
place for people who are dying. Medicine prescribes boundaries of how

its patients are supposed to think about who they are, and thus how they are to accept being treated.[36] Patients who are dying have no place within these boundaries. In Bérubé's terms, their feelings are not narratable as stories that institutional medicine can recognize. Patients who deny they are dying are thus not "in denial." On the contrary, they are being considerate enough to collude in medicine's denying them a place.

Kramer illustrates medical denial in a story about her aunt, who has just had exploratory abdominal surgery. The medical judgment is that "nothing could be done." This phrase is given literal meaning during her aunt's postsurgical care. Kramer retells the story as her aunt told it to her:

It was late in the evening, and the staff was efficiently bustling around her bed setting up an automatic dispenser for pain control drugs. (The theory behind these devices is that they give patients more autonomy by allowing them to pace their own medications: the push of a button dispenses small doses of the total prescription.) Everything was in place, the staff went away, and my aunt was left to ride the roller-coaster of her own thoughts, but the first time she pushed the button, the machine, to use her words, "blew up."

This event produced prompt and intense activity. "Do you know," she said, "I had six of them in there—a whole crowd of people, some of them on their hands and knees—all trying to fix the machine. They seemed to take an eternity." (When we are in great pain like this, eternity has a way of opening up under us, and over us, and to the side of us.) In the end, the machine was deemed impossible to repair, and the crowd of people left, wheeling it with them, leaving my aunt alone. "They were all totally avoiding me," she said. "It made me feel so alone, so utterly alone. I felt as though I must be the only person this had ever happened to."

After a while a nurse came in, all efficient and professional with a questionnaire. This was presumably a standard questionnaire to establish a course of pain control. My aunt said, "You'll never guess what the first question was: 'What do you perceive to be the source of your pain?'" My aunt felt as though she had been caught in an absurdist play. How could the nurse not see? There's always physical pain after this kind of surgery. There's always emotional and psychological pain when treatments fail.

But here the thread of mortality that is within all of us, all our lives, was emerging and becoming clearly apparent in her. Everyone in the room knew it was so. But once the technology broke down, from my aunt's point of view, that particular group of health care professionals was left resourceless. As my aunt said, "No one made eye contact with me. No one reached out to touch me." (1)

Kramer responds to her aunt's story with a Stoic question: "What do I perceive to be the source of *my* pain about all this?" (4) That question can be answered only in a dialogical context. Although the palliative care movement has affected some medical practices, Kramer wonders how much has changed. She thinks of the memo she received from the cancer center where she was treated. The news that their treatments could no longer arrest the spread of cancer was phrased as "Patient failed to respond to treatments" (4). This misrepresents who, or what, failed—the patient is blamed for the treatment's failure. But the more insidious representation is to frame dying as a failure. The entire cancer center behaves like the six professionals in her aunt's hospital room. When they can't fix the machine, they all leave, avoiding— and in the cancer center's note, blaming—the dying woman. Avoiding their patient, they avoid the inevitability of death as part of the ecology of life.

"How can the medical staff appear so resourceless in the face of something that happens again and again?" Kramer asks. She realizes that the staff cannot respond because her aunt's dying is not narratable in any terms they consider acceptable for use by medical professionals. Her aunt's suffering becomes invisible, just as Kramer becomes invisible; she is another of those who have "failed," in her cancer center's description. Once the center has run out of chemo and radiation protocols, they have no other narrative, so Kramer's aunt ceases to be narratable.[37] Kramer, however, has other narratives available; like Williams, she's a naturalist. Her own answer to her question of why the staff appears so resourceless is "We lack an ability to think of death in ecological terms" (4).

To help us begin to think ecologically and generously, Kramer takes us into a swamp.

At one time in the past, I was involved in biological fieldwork. I hiked through tropical rain forests, waded in rivers, and slogged through lots of swamps. There's nothing like a swamp to give you a firsthand look at parts of the ecosystem.

The word *ecology* comes from the Greek root meaning "house." Most of us have probably lived in houses and know well that they constantly need repair. If you wade out into a swamp, step by step you stir up and move through one of the

foundations of our ecological house. You enter an earthy, fluid confluence of decay. Because the oxygen level in the water is low, the process of decay is slow and
very evident. That's what makes a swamp a good place to think about death. But
amid this decay, the swamp is a nurturing habitat for hundreds of life forms. For
whether we like it or not, death is the process that helps keep the ecosystem reno-
vated. It's the universal composter. In this sense, death is very much part of an
endless recovery model. An endless process of renewal. (4)

Marcus Aurelius would love this story. He advocated seeing things
just as they are (see ix.29: "Nothing but phlegm and mucus"), and the
decay in Kramer's swamp would have furnished him with numerous
metaphors. "Condition of the Body: *decaying*," (ii.16), he wrote. Marcus would have reminded us that those rotting beings remain part
of what he would call the *logos*, but he might have liked calling it
Kramer's "universal composter" (cf. ix.35). Death for Marcus is not destruction but only part of what Kramer calls "an endless recovery
model." Heraclitus made fire his metaphor for renewal through
change; the swamp is even better. "All substance is soon absorbed into
nature . . . all trace of them both soon covered over by time" (vii.10).

Marcus writes so much about the eternal harmony because as he
dealt with rebellions within the Roman Empire and barbarian wars
on its borders, he saw as much death and destruction as a contemporary oncologist sees. Through all that horror, Marcus managed to keep
the thought of universal harmony before him, a harmony that includes death's integral part in life. He remained able to offer consolation to the dying. The medical professionals who can't look Kramer's
aunt in the eye have lost their sense of death's harmony. They have no
consolation to offer, so they cannot allow themselves to perceive a need
for consolation.

Kramer's aunt, because she is dying, becomes a human absence, to
be managed at a distance by machines and questionnaires. Kramer
describes how the staff's response to her aunt was typical of others'
treatment:

But I am still haunted by the voices of cancer patients: "They are afraid to touch
me." Or, "They touch me as if I'm already dead." Or, "Most of the time they
look right through me." Or, "I can't tell one from another; they never introduce
themselves." Sometimes I think there's a regulation that we are not allowed to be
real people. Sometimes I think professionalism is a handicap we all labor under.

On really bad days, I have had the urge to tap on the shoulder of a particular nurse or doctor or technician and shout, "Hey! Is anybody in there?" (5)

When Kramer offers observations like these to medical students, they throw up their hands and complain that it's too much to ask of them.[38] "What?" Kramer replies rhetorically, "Just to be able to look someone in the eye?" (5), which takes us all the way back to Peschel and Mr. B in chapter 1. Generosity begins with being able to look someone in the eye.

I was editor of the series of journal articles in which Kramer's essay was published, and what generated the most controversy was her bringing her ecological vision of illness and death down to the level of personal decisions about treatment for cancer:

In the "battle" to prolong our lives as individuals, medical research has been given the green light to do whatever it takes to keep death at bay. Consequently, as a woman with breast cancer, I have been offered treatments that are incompatible with the function and spirit of the ecosystem. I've been offered radiotherapy and the diagnostic tools of nuclear medicine, extensions of a larger nuclear industry that threatens widespread environmental damage in the form of radiation. If anything is capable of dousing the light of the ecosystem for good, it's probably elevated levels of radiation from the uranium cycle. I've been offered chemotherapy, a heavy-duty version of the "Better Living through Chemistry" campaign. That campaign has unleashed thousands of tons of human-made chemicals into the environment in this century. (4)

Several medical and ethics professionals who were asked to referee the acceptability of Kramer's manuscript for publication wanted to cut this passage. Suggestions that patients should even consider refusing treatment on ecological grounds—counseling noncompliance, raising questions about the environmental ethics of medicine—were not acceptable for publication in a clinical ethics journal.

Kramer was raising at least two issues that were too much of a Pandora's box (in the language of chapter 1) for publication. The issues of her aunt's abandonment and of medicine's denial of death were all right to raise; those fell into the sphere of legitimate controversy. But the suggestion that medical treatments should be rejected if incompatible with the good of the ecosystem was not up for discussion. Behind that issue is the larger question of Brookes's health ecology. Kramer's implication that she refused "treatments that are incompatible with the ecosystem" radicalizes what Brookes writes. She affirms Brookes's core insight: "When one person falls ill or stays healthy, the entire universe is involved." She adds the recognition that life needs each of us to die; it's our last, generous service.

Kramer may approach death like Marcus Aurelius, but she approaches medicine in the spirit of Levinas. She understands herself as chosen by cancer; she is the first to hear the call. Her cancer is her family's cancer, and that circle expands. Kramer feels herself to be responsible for everything, most of all for the fate of others. In the swamp, seeing decay face to face and realizing her place in that harmony, she discovers "that the death of the other has priority over your own and over your life," as Levinas puts it.[39] Levinas's examples involve one person responding to the need of another person: "To throw yourself into the water to save someone, without knowing how to swim, is to go toward the other wholly; without holding back of oneself" (127). Kramer throws herself in to save not any specific other person, but the life that she finds in the swamp, the same life that Williams finds in the desert. Swamp and desert are the "home" that life needs. Whatever violates the home cannot heal. Kramer refuses treatments, or implies she might, because medical use of chemicals that are toxic to the earth contradicts an ecological understanding of life. Like Williams, she insists that a whole new contract be drawn up, a contract generous to life.

Kramer makes illness a moral occasion to ask what the human home is, and how we hurt ourselves when we fail to understand death as part of the truth of this home. She asks whether medicine as we know it is keeping up repairs on this home, or whether it has become part of what's risking "dousing the light of the ecosystem for good" (4). Her primary concern is not if she lives or dies—death is only a question of when, and in her Stoic way, she perceives the greater harmony.

Kramer's generosity is to be more concerned with the future of the home, the swamp, than with herself. This concern depends on her dialogical insight that she exists only as part of the home. "When I look at the big picture," she says, "I have to ask: what's the use of being a survivor if you've got nowhere to go home to" (5).

Levinas expands the sense of "Thou shall not kill" to include whatever might harm the other in any way, thus making himself wholly responsible.[40] Similarly, Kramer takes the medical injunction "First, do no harm" and extends it beyond the individual physician's responsibility to individual patients to the ecology of life that sustains those patients by being their home.[41] Those who advised against publication of her essay could not admit that ecological recognition into the conversation; they denied the narratability of the ecology of illness. Kramer pushed the horizon of what is ethical too far.

"Are we so afraid of seeing our own reflection?" she asks at the end of her essay. "What *are* we afraid of?" (5)

Moral Nonfiction

I have described how ill and disabled people seek to create more generous representations of themselves and their conditions; how the ill seek to sustain their participation and to make society more generous in the forms of participation that it values; and finally the generosity of expanding personal health to health ecology. The generosity of the ill goes beyond these issues, but this discussion makes the point that the ill are remoralizing illness and its treatment.

If the stories I tell in this book need a label, I call them moral nonfiction, a category best described by Levinas: "it makes a demand on me." The written text shows the reader a face that "looks at me and calls to me. It lays claim to me. What does it ask? Not to leave it alone. An answer: here I am."[42] The moral moment is when the text calls on the reader—on *me*—just as the patient calls on those who offer care. The here-I-am of the writer is a generous offering of self as witness. This generosity calls for a response of here-I-am from the reader. Levinas says that the face of the other obligates me not to abandon them. In turn, a reader may be obligated not to allow a story to end there. The dialogue of author and reader is the beginning of other dialogues: in the multiple sites where medicine is offered and received, where care is given, and where healing occurs.

CHAPTER FOUR

Physicians' Generosity

I N the previous chapter ill people act generously without doctors, and occasionally in spite of doctors. But many ill people, when they are patients, harbor an intuition that their physicians know aspects of their suffering as no one else can. Among all the words of others that shape an ill person, the physician's words have particular significance—if those words are spoken *to* the person who happens to be a patient, not *about* the patient who contains a disease. The patient's desire for a human relationship with a physician is expressed with wit and generosity by Anatole Broyard:

Thus the hero's words about himself are structured under the continuous influence of someone else's words about him.
MIKHAIL BAKHTIN

Marja [his wife] and I realized that we wanted to be closer to the people with whom we worked, that if we didn't move closer we might end up moving much farther away.
DAVID HILFIKER

88

I have a wistful desire for our relationship to be beautiful in some way that I can't quite identify. . . . Just as he orders blood tests and bone scans of my body, I'd like my doctor to scan *me*, to grope for my spirit as well as my prostate. . . . I would also like a doctor who *enjoyed* me. I want to be a good story for him, to give him some of my art in exchange for his. . . . There should be a place where our respective superiorities could meet and frolic together.[1]

Broyard emphasizes the modesty of his desire; he does not want his doctor to stop being a doctor or lose "his technical posture." Broyard does not expect his doctor to love him, but he does want to be known in his singularity: "I would also like to think of him as going through my character, as he goes through my flesh, for each man is ill in his own way" (44).

Some patients enjoy relationships like the one Broyard wants, either because they find the right doctor or because they take extraordinary steps. I met a man who had undergone a bone marrow transplant for leukemia, a procedure that involves prolonged hospitalization in isolation (due to induced immune suppression) with horrific side-effects of treatment. In his room at a major medical center he set up a toy basketball hoop, and he required any physician who came into the room to take a foul shot before he'd talk to him. Some doctors thought he was kidding. He wasn't. They shot a basket, then talked. He was a self-described "medical entrepreneur" who had worked with doctors and medical institutions for years before he became a patient. He knew how far he could push. He created Broyard's space of mutual frolic by mandating those moments of taking the foul shot, thereby changing the spirit in which doctor and patient returned to other matters. This patient is the exception. Most end up like Evan Handler, discussed in chapter 3: better advised to find a physician they can use and go elsewhere to talk about healing.

This chapter reflects on stories by physicians who want what Broyard wants: for their relationships with their patients to be beautiful in some way. I choose four physicians—Abraham Verghese, Rafael Campo, Lori Alvord, and David Hilfiker—who are established in their profession but are young as the life span goes; the oldest is late middle-aged. These doctors reached their career potential long after physicians regularly made house calls, and long enough after the sky's-the-limit medical boom of the 1960s and 1970s, when the professional power of medicine may have enjoyed its historical zenith. Their medical world is epitomized by two phenomena that became prominent in the 1980s: managed care and AIDS.

Physicians are still afforded considerable prestige and rewards, but during the last twenty-five years their everyday work has been increasingly circumscribed, often not so subtly, by an administration whose training and accountability are nonmedical. This corporate and government bureaucracy conceives care as a quantity of goods and services to be allocated as scarce resources and/or commodities. The circumscription of physician autonomy effected by managed care is exacerbated by the uncertainty of the AIDS pandemic, which has stretched the limits of medicine's capacity to care and become a metaphor of the limits of medical power, or hubris, to control disease.

The physicians who lend their stories to this chapter began their careers when medicine faced a disease that was undiagnosed, deadly, and wholly outside its control. Multiple personal and professional ethical questions were raised by the effect of AIDS on selective groups: first gay men, then the inner-city poor. Physicians had to think about the limits of their obligations to *these* patients; offering treatment was believed to be physically dangerous due to risk of infection; issues of blaming patients for "lifestyle choices" were inescapable. AIDS remains a crisis of medical uncertainty that underscores the effects of social marginalization on risk of disease and access to care. This crisis occurred at the same moment that society was questioning medical costs and demanding restraint. These four doctors represent a physician cohort that could not learn all they need to know from the example and experience of their mentors. They continue to have to work out, in new conditions of practice, how to be the professionals they want to be.

Abraham Verghese expresses a younger physician's sense of his profession having lost a fundamental part of its moral identity:

My physician-uncle in India told me how, as a young doctor, he had gone more than once into a hushed house where an entire household had bolted, abandoning their loved one because of smallpox. The unfortunate patient, covered with pustules, lay comatose on a mat on the floor, the rice and barley water that had been left beside him now crawling with ants. My uncle had hired a ricksha, loaded the patient on it and taken him to the communicable disease hospital. In the days to come, my uncle waited for the pustules to appear on his own skin, for the rigors and chills to commence. He had been lucky.

American medicine by the 1970s and 1980s was different. The new icons included the Porsche Targa, not designed for house calls. Personal risk had all but disappeared. Professional liability had taken its place. Evening clinics were anathema. In its place were doc-in-the-box centers, emergency rooms, answering services, beepers, cross-coverage and cellular phones. Money was the obvious and very visible reward for being a physician. Lifestyle was a key factor in the decision to become a doctor and the choice of specialties. . . . Doctors were reimbursed generously for doing, but not for thinking.[2]

This contrast does not recommend nostalgia for the good old days of exposure to life-threatening risk. Verghese, whose fears of being infected with HIV are described later in this chapter, is thankful not to be called to do what his uncle did. Nonetheless, he takes seriously what is lost by no longer having to do that. A physician like his uncle was a healing presence because he had the aura of one who risks his life for his patients. When he risked his body, he reminded himself and his community what it meant to be a physician. Verghese asks how to sustain that moral commitment.

Each of these physicians works to get over having been demoralized by medical training and conditions of practice. Each seeks remoralization through becoming the storyteller that Broyard wants his physician to be. As physician-writers, they show that a dialogical medicine is possible. Each understands how much is at stake in creating dialogue.

The task and dilemma of the physician as storyteller can be introduced by philosopher Alasdair MacIntyre's influential description of storytelling:

> [M]an is in his actions and practice, as well as in his fictions, essentially a storytelling animal. He . . . becomes through his history a teller of stories that aspire to truth. But the key question for men is not about their own authorship; I can only answer the question, "What am I to do?" if I can answer the prior question "Of what story or stories do I find myself a part?" We enter human society, that is, with one or more imputed characters—roles into which we have been drafted—and we have to learn what they are in order to be able to understand how others respond to us and how our responses to them are apt to be construed.[3]

The physicians I discuss in this chapter might consider themselves well represented by the first part of MacIntyre's argument. Their storytelling aspires to tell a truth about illness, suffering, and medical care. Each of the physicians in this chapter faces constant situations that require asking, "What am I to do?" and each needs to tell his or her stories in order to answer the complementary question that MacIntyre states so well: "Of what story or stories do I find myself a part?" Having posed that question, MacIntyre is less useful describing how these physicians respond to it.

All of these physicians have a problem that MacIntyre does not immediately recognize.[4] All, as MacIntyre says, find themselves with an imputed character, a role or roles into which they have been drafted, but all feel misrepresented by that role. All resist being responded to as that imputed character. All tell stories to get themselves *out of* at least one of the stories of which they are part. Getting out of an old story requires telling a new one, but all these physicians find that no adequate story is culturally ready-made.[5] A new story—a new possibility of being a physician—has to be created.

A new story is necessary because the conditions of medical practice have changed, and because these physicians bring a heightened self-awareness to their work. Each, by virtue of one or more personal or professional qualities, feels marginal either to medicine or to society as a whole. Some marginalities, including ethnicity and sexual orientation, could be called demographic. These marginalities instigate a questioning of received values: all four physicians wonder from whom they are to receive which values.

These physicians' sense of personal marginality exacerbates their sensitivity to a generalized medical crisis over what Charles Taylor calls *hypergoods*. Hypergoods are "higher-order goods," that is, "goods which are not only incomparably more important than others but provide the standpoint from which these [other goods] must be weighed, judged, decided upon."[6] Taylor describes hypergoods as "a set of ends or demands which . . . override and allow us to judge others [i.e., other competing goods]" (63). He immediately notes that people often do not share the same hypergoods. People's own hypergoods are so embedded in their being that they have difficulty imagining how other people could find their hypergoods to be compelling. Thus dialogue breaks down, and hypergoods—which are necessary to organize choices at a lower level—are "generally a source of conflict" (64).

An earlier generation of physicians, if asked what hypergood guided their work, might have felt it sufficient to answer, "Medicine." Medicine was imagined as a unity of knowledge, fraternity, and value that could provide a guide. Verghese's physician uncle might have claimed medicine as his hypergood and felt enough had been said. Professional medicine in the age of managed care and AIDS is less sure of its hypergoods; consequently, fragmentation over hypergoods makes appeal to some unified *medicine* increasingly tenuous. A sense of personal marginality heightens this fragmentation. Physicians who see their own marginalities reflected in their patients—and who learn from their patients how they themselves are marginal, in ways they had not realized—have no stable hypergoods that can order the choices they make in their lives and work. They have to think through what their values are, and writing is a medium of that thought.

These physicians' writing is animated by their uncertainty about which story or stories they *ought* to be part of, which stories they *resist* being part of, and what story they may have to create as the story they *do* want to be part of. Each writes in order to discover; discovery happens through crafting his or her story, and that process continues as each book ends. These searches take place in dialogue, since individual stories can only be told in multiple relations of *with:* with patients, with family, with colleagues and teachers. These physicians survive by doing what Broyard (44) wants his doctors to do: they brood on their patients, and that is indistinguishable from brooding on themselves. They bond with their sickest patients' uncertainty as to what story their lives have made them part of and what values direct those lives. These physicians' generosity is embodied in their openness to their patients' suffering that exceeds their pain and disease.[7]

PHYSICIANS' DEMORALIZATION

These four physicians tell a collective story of how medical training and practice demoralize them. Rafael Campo describes the demoralization of his early career as a volatile combination of personal history and institutional milieu. As a medical resident Campo does work that most would consider morally admirable: like Verghese, he treats patients who have AIDS in the early days of the epidemic. But he treats them without caring for them. He meets their basic medical needs but rejects their humanity. Campo feels overwhelmed, and he withdraws. He describes how he regards one patient:

He was little more than a disgusting chore to me, something akin to mopping up a stubbornly grimy floor. In my view, each new hospitalization he had required, thickening his chart as if only to make it heavier for me to lug back and forth from medical records, was a waste of already scarce public health dollars.[8]

Campo does exactly what Verghese describes contemporary physicians being encouraged to do: he minimizes thinking. He does so as "one of my intern's strategies for conserving energy" (37). Campo is caught between his hospital's need for billable procedures and society's preference for having people taken care of elsewhere and as cheaply as possible.

The energy he conserves is negative, feeding his worst impulses at increasing personal cost: "I was becoming what in my most frightened moments I had always dreamed of becoming, another instrument of precise algorithms, a sharp metal tool by which the exact distance from health to disease could be calculated to within three decimal places" (113). Campo's confessional vehemence is singular, but his observation that medicine taught him to be what he feared becoming is shared by others.

Lori Alvord writes of having to "unlearn" much of what her medical training taught her.[9] She criticizes medicine for the same reasons expressed by Anatole Broyard, Evan Handler, and Vanessa Kramer:

Now more than ever, patients themselves feel removed and forgotten, powerless in the face of the institutions that were created to help them. In many ways modern medicine has become a one-way system—from physicians to patient. Physicians do the directing, talking at their patients. The other direction, the listening on the part of the physician, is becoming lost. Patients . . . want to feel like more than a set of organs and bones, nerves and blood, and participate in the process of restoring their bodies to health. (2)

In the distortion of relationships that medical practice perpetrates, "both patients and physicians suffer" (2). Alvord understands this suffering as the result of medicine forgetting what her Native American traditions insist she remember: "Everything in life is connected." Remoralization requires "a medicine that does not isolate but connects" (3). Before considering the subtle nature of this connection, a final dimension of demoralization needs to be added.

The four physicians discussed in this chapter construct their lives and careers around a geographic journey. Of these, Verghese's journey is the most geographically extensive, taking him from Africa, where he was born and did his early medical training, to the United States, then to India (his family's country of origin) for medical school, and finally back to America. Campo's journey is the most metaphoric. He comes not by birth but by culture and spirit from Cuba, his parents' home country. Cuba remains Campo's imaginary homeland, the locus of his poetic imagination. It is where his identity begins, although he has never been there.[10] Alvord's journey is from the Navajo reservations of the Four Corners area of New Mexico to the universities (Dartmouth and Stanford) where she becomes a surgeon and eventually teaches and practices surgery. Our fourth physician, David Hilfiker, moves from medical practice with middle-class patients in rural Minnesota to inner-city Washington, D.C., to care for the poorest and most underserved patients.[11]

Verghese, in the long quotation earlier in this chapter, writes that lifestyle was becoming the key determinant in physicians' choices of specialty. Hilfiker presents medicine as both reflecting and exacerbating the gulf between those who can afford to think of their lives as a lifestyle and those who barely survive in conditions that the first group would find unimaginable.[12] Many of his patients have diseases that people with regular incomes, and the housing and diet that go with those incomes, rarely would be at risk for. Those of his patients who have diseases that can affect anyone live in conditions that generate complications and worse prognoses. Poverty prevents people from being treated and denies them the resources necessary to comply with treatment; a patient cannot take medication with meals if regular meals are not part of life.

Hilfiker sees medicine's demoralization beginning in its institutionalized incomprehension of what illness means in circumstances when disease is no longer "a distinct phenomenon that could be treated in and of itself."[13] His assessment of how the medical profession has lost its own moral grounds begins with its deprecation of his work, which he calls "poverty medicine":

> There is no [medical school] curriculum for poverty medicine: no one teaches "The Art of Medical Decision Making With Limited Funds" or "Medical Compromise with Cultural Strictures." Medical practice in a community of poor people often seems a solitary specialty without research, common cause, or shared experience. I and my few partners are isolated professionally, with no way even to assess our own record. . . . As a physician for the poor, I know there will be no "professional advancement." The bottom rung of the ladder is the same as the top rung: working as a clinic doctor, seeing patients day-to-day. (213)

Hilfiker does not want professional recognition for himself; instead, professional recognition of poverty medicine would acknowledge the patients who are now systematically excluded.

Demoralization in poverty medicine is the daily need for "almost indecent compromise of professional standards" (213). The compromises of treatment that Hilfiker is forced to make because of lack of resources are then held against him as reasons he should not be practicing where he is. After a lecture Hilfiker gives at a university medical school, a professor asks him whether he doesn't think he is wasting his professional education: "It seems to me that your job might better be done by a social worker or nurse practitioner, while you used your talents more effectively elsewhere." Hilfiker does not take offense. He has an extraordinary dialogical capacity to recognize the rationality of any stance, given where it comes from. He has his own self-doubts about when he might "get to the point where I am unqualified to be a 'real doctor'" (212).

But the professor does not seem to consider the alternative that his question presupposes: Hilfiker leaving his patients with no physician at all. This abandonment is troubling not necessarily because the quality of treatment in the clinic would get worse. Given the diminished conditions that Hilfiker works in, possibly a nurse practitioner could exercise a comparable level of clinical judgment and intervention skill, and these instrumental outcomes are all the professor counts as significant. Conversely, Hilfiker understands that a considerable part of his value to his patients is symbolic. A doctor is more than a set of skills. A doctor is a status, and the presence of that status conveys social inclusion; patients attended by a doctor have not been abandoned. Hilfiker knows that by being present as a doctor in his inner-city clinic, he embodies a connection between the medicine of those who have lifestyles and the lives of those who are most marginalized. Verghese's uncle did not exercise any particular medical skills when he hauled his smallpox-infected patients out of their houses; that, too, was not a good use of his professional training. But it was essential that he do this himself, to remind everyone who a doctor is.

Hilfiker cannot offer his patients what he took for granted in his Minnesota practice: prompt access to specialist referral, testing, or inpatient admission. Reflecting on what he *can* offer, he concludes: "I can offer myself and my presence as a healer. The recent tide of technological medicine has tended to erode our understanding of the fundamental imperative for any physician—to be a healing presence" (227). The demoralization of medicine means the loss of that healing presence. This loss is expressed in how different medical activities and specialties are allocated rewards, time, and physical space. Who gets how much of these is no longer organized according to the hypervalue that the physician's presence, in itself, can be healing.

Hilfiker concludes that mainstream medicine needs poverty medicine to recollect its calling: "to offer unconditional acceptance of the patient's being; to clarify (without judgment) the cause of the illness; to honor the pain, to recognize the fear, and to hold on to the hope" (228). Those goals define the remoralization of medicine.

The question that Alvord, Campo, Hilfiker, and Verghese all face is how to realize these goals in their moment-by-moment interactions with their patients. They are Stoic in asking what it is that they can control. They wonder what their moral character depends on. They are dialogical in thinking first of how they act toward others. The practice of generosity—not the advance of science or the increase of billable services, but a physician's version of health ecology—is the hypergood that organizes the stories they want their lives to be part of.

Encountering the Other, Outside and Inside

A single theme that organizes the diffuse work of these four physicians is expressed by the title of Rafael Campo's first book of poetry: *The Other Man Was Me*.[14] Each of these physicians is concerned with how to encounter patients who are radically different in the material, intellectual, and spiritual conditions of their lives. They differ in the choices that express their values and hypergoods. As each physician encounters the otherness of his or her patients, the relationship to the other who is outside mirrors an internal relation of otherness between parts of the self. The problem—very much a clinical problem, in these physicians' judgment—is how to be generous toward the other. Each learns that it is difficult, maybe impossible, to be any more generous to the other outside than you are generous to the other inside.

Verghese tracks his progress from taking a literary interest in his patients to seeing his problems reflected in theirs. This shift makes him better able to help and heal. He begins wanting to be the kind of doctor whom Broyard wants. He describes letting his patients be good stories for him: "I was fascinated by the voyage that had brought them to my clinic door. The anecdotes they told me lingered in my mind and became the way I identified them."[15] He writes these stories down, keeping a journal that becomes increasingly important to him. He self-consciously looks forward to the visits of a patient with whom he can readily identify: a man his age, heterosexual, infected with HIV by a blood transfusion to treat his hemophilia. "I would anticipate his visits, looking forward to drawing him out," Verghese writes. "In learning about him it seemed I was learning about myself" (269).

But Verghese soon realizes that his patients are and will remain

other to him. Their otherness only begins in differences of their birth-
place, education, and sexual orientation (most of his patients are gay;
he isn't). The deepest divide is sickness. His patients, diagnosed as
having AIDS when the disease had just been named and could not be
treated, remain on the other side of a divide he crosses only in recur-
ring dreams of being infected. Verghese's initial interest in keeping a
journal of favorite patient anecdotes could turn him into another phy-
sician-as-literary-spectator. The terror of his dreams shows him the
truth of the story he is part of, the story he must offer to witness in his
writing as well as in his medical work.

> The dream recurred so often—always in a different form—I thought of it as the
> "infection" dream. [He describes the dream, to the moment when he is told his
> blood test for the presence of HIV is positive.] "Nooooo!" I screamed. I wept and
> said it was a mistake, but she shook her head, a little amused by my histrionics,
> as if one should be able to take this sort of news in one's stride—particularly a
> *medical* man. . . .
>
>   I woke in a cold sweat. Each time I had this dream, I immediately recalled the
> last time I had broken the news of a positive test to a young man. I remembered
> my concern, my empathy, my encouraging and supportive tone, as if to say,
> "Don't worry, I know what you are going through, and it will be all right." But a
> dream like this made me feel like I had no idea what I was saying. In my waking
> hours I never understood the absolute terror of finding out you have HIV; in my
> dreams I understood all too well. (302–3)

Verghese can brood with his patients, just as Broyard wants a physician who will brood with him. He can even love and suffer with his
patients, which is more than Broyard felt he could ask for. But perhaps
most important, Verghese realizes that he has no idea what his patients
are going through; he knows the distance of their otherness. He also
realizes that his ability to care for them as their doctor depends on how
he balances the dialogical closeness of their relationship—the existence of each on the boundary with the other—against what his consciousness can never merge with: those parts of his patients' lives that
will always remain other to him, but that command his respect all the
more because they are other.

Verghese is explicit about the interdependence between his patients' otherness and his own sense of not belonging: "There was an
obvious parallel: society considered [his gay patients who have AIDS]

alien and much of their life was spent faking conformity; in my case my Green Card labeled me as a "'resident alien'" (51). He describes a confrontation with a pharmacist who had violated confidentiality about a patient with AIDS; in their heated exchange, Verghese hears himself being called a "foreign doctor." Later his wife asks him if the pharmacist actually said that, or if Verghese felt "as if he said it." He admits the latter (248). That evening Verghese studies a map of the United States, asking himself, "Was there some place in the country where I could walk around anonymously, where I could blend in completely with a community, be undistinguished by appearance, accent or speech?" (249).[16] He crafts a story in which his encounters with his patients, the other outside, are informed and enhanced by his sense of being alien in his foreignness, the other inside. Verghese's writing is anything but the after-hours diversion of a physician expressing his artistic side. His medical practice and his life depend on the story he creates.

Rafael Campo feels divided not only between geographical origins, but also between sexual and professional identities. I heard Campo begin a conference lecture by joking that when he arrived at Harvard Medical School as a student, what most upset people about him was not that he was Cuban, nor that he was gay, but that he was—and here Campo's voice rises to mock indignation—a poet!

At the time Campo finishes Harvard and begins his medical residency, he does not imagine learning about himself from his patients. He trains himself not only in distancing himself from them but even in contempt, which he evokes with chilling confessional honesty:

Each bone marrow biopsy, each rectal exam, each electrocardioversion I performed seemed only to compound the indignity of it all. I watched with detachment at the end of so many lives, as unmoved and bored as if I were taking out the garbage. In the cold glare of my new secular reasoning, without their humanity, without even their souls, such patients became unmissable targets for the senseless blame I had once felt and now deflected onto others. . . .

I frequently reminded myself that I was not among them, that I was somehow different. Internally I accused them of a quasi-religious checklist of crimes of which I believed myself to be innocent. They were promiscuous, while I was monogamous. They were stupid, stupid enough to get infected, while I was clever. They were fornicators, while I loved another man. They were failures; I, a

young graduate of Amherst College and Harvard Medical School, was at a pinna-
cle of achievement and still full of promise. They fretted about the fates of their
souls, while I knew there was nothing after this life. They would allow themselves to be judged by God, while I judged them haughtily.[17]

With this bitter logic he rejects his "fundamental human bond with
such patients" (53).

Campo does not come to this way of thinking on his own. Medical
school crystallizes his most destructive self-doubts and prepares him
to turn these against his patients. Early in his training he begins to believe "that identity was somehow intertwined with immunity" (182),
and that immunity is conferred by knowing who one is. He idealizes
the stable, unified identity of the white heterosexual male who, Campo
imagines, is secure in the knowledge that the story he is part of was
written expressly for a person like himself. The final link in this unhappy syllogism is what Campo calls "a method for pathologizing myself" and confirming "that I did not belong. . . . That I was *unhealthy*"
(183). Feeling himself to be unhealthy, Campo can imagine no health
in his patients. His hostility to the other who is inside is projected
against the other outside.

Campo is pulled out of this spiral by a risk of becoming one of those
patients. While he is attempting to start an IV on a patient who has
AIDS, the man suddenly flails about, and Campo is stuck with the
same needle he had been inserting into the man's vein. What follows is
a moral epiphany:

The rent in my skin was only two or three millimeters in size, though the small
amount of blood that had fanned out in the subcutaneous tissue made a dusky red
spot that was alarmingly much bigger, maybe a centimeter or so. I squeezed out
whatever blood I could, not knowing whether the drop or two I was able to express was mine or his, or mine mixed with his. I changed my scrub pants in one
of the deserted hallways of the labyrinthine OR, the dried blood that had soaked
in pulling at the hair on my thigh as I shucked them off, not caring if a stray or-
derly or scrub nurse happened to spy me undressed: I finally knew how human I
was, I was made acutely aware in one terrible moment that all any of us has in
the world is the same body.

[W]hat was happening to me in the utility closet felt like an opening, a revela-
tion, a chance for survival. . . . Perhaps in the mixing of my blood with another
person's, I could learn the true meaning of forgiveness. (59–61)

Campo thus joins Schweitzer's fellowship of those who bear the mark of pain. He has been a member for a long time, but unable to claim his membership. The needle-stick allows Campo to name the pain he has felt in so many aspects of his life and to give it positive purpose. A conflicted Catholic, he makes peace with a faith that he can now use as a poetic to express his moral imagination:

Even the most despised and isolated of patients has someone to whom he can turn, one who truly does have the power to heal, a hope that is the source of all poems. The terrifying needle-stick is just a reminder, the bearded chaplain on his rounds exudes a kind of comfort, the hideous skin lesion becomes the glorious imprint of God's touch. Today I see that the handsome nurse carrying away feces in a bedpan is an angel; the quiet glance we exchange is the meaning of life. (61–62)

The needle-stick is one of a series of recognitions that bring Campo into a new self-acceptance and a new relationship with his patients. His clear lesson to physicians is that they cannot treat their patients any better than they treat themselves, and medical school was all too fertile a ground for his self-doubts to turn punitive. Medicine's demoralization is reflected in how readily a hospital could capitalize, literally, on the young resident's punitive feelings toward himself and his patients. Campo changes because some latent generosity within him finds expression, not because his institution or senior mentors lead him to change.

Campo's patients remain other to him, but this otherness is who they are as people; it's the otherness that makes dialogue possible. Campo is no longer alienated from their otherness. Then he meets Manuel, a patient who "bluntly" describes his attempts to contract HIV by having anonymous sex with multiple partners. " I could barely hide my fast-rising disgust and rage," Campo recalls, "while a less emotional part of me bristled with disbelief." Manuel keeps talking, "perhaps sensing some remnant in me that was still capable of listening" (185).

Campo's encounter with Manuel recapitulates the dialogical relationship: the other person is first heard as speaking from some unimaginable moral universe, but his speech crystallizes into an imaginable life that expands the moral imagination of the listener. The speaker gradually becomes not only plausible but, while still other, honorable in that otherness.

He wanted to die, he said, because he could not stand to wipe up another lover's diarrhea from the floor in a dining room where they had once shared meals with other friends long since dead of AIDS; he could not bear another message from his mother on his answering machine wondering whether he was still alive, imploring him to leave San Francisco and return to their church in the Central Valley. He had come to believe that HIV infection was as inevitable as seeing his own face in the mirror when he shaved in the morning, as much a part of his life as attending memorial services and reading the obituaries. He would not let himself become another victim, he said, but rather would face his destiny with courage. He paused and looked me straight in the eye.

I felt a weight beginning to shift in my chest, as though a new passageway were being pried open. . . . My pat theories about health and disease ran away from me as I stared back into his unclouded face. (185–86)

Campo's acceptance of Manuel is not a bonding. The dialogical morality of their encounter lies in Manuel continuing to tell his story in the face of Campo's initial reaction, and Campo, at least "some remnant" in him, continuing to listen to this intolerable story.[18] To paraphrase the title of Campo's book of poetry, the other man is *not* me, but the other man shares enough *with* me to remind me that I exist on the boundary between us. With different experiences, in different circumstances, the other man could be me.

David Hilfiker's choice not only to care for the poor but to live among them is grounded in his religious faith, that "each of us is inextricably bound to—indeed, tangled up with—the pain of the poor," with whom we share a "common community."[19] Yet Hilfiker emphasizes the eternal gulf between himself as host and his guests. He speaks of the need for *identification* with the poor, giving this phrase a particular meaning, for his *identification* is not being *identical with*. What he means by identification begins with recognizing the fundamental difference between people whose lives have been shaped by poverty and those like himself and most of his readers. Hilfiker explains this difference:

There are privileges of birth and up-bringing I could never renounce, even if I wanted to. I could give away all of my money, but none of my education. No matter how poor I became, I would always have the possibility of returning to the mainstream and beginning again. . . . And were all of these [possibilities which Hilfiker has detailed] taken away, I would still have a lifelong sense of entitlement to fall back on, far stronger than any entitlement program a government has ever conceived. I would have the secure psychological background of a childhood valued by parents, of trust in stable relationships, of confidence that I was able to handle whatever came to me in life. No matter what happens to me in the future, I will never share the experience of growing up poor and powerless within the abusive environment of the inner city. . . .

The landscape of poverty is inaccessible to most of us. We can barely imagine the scenery. (78–79)

Hilfiker's ideal of identification with the poor is a willed and learned ability to imagine what effect any attitude or action or policy will have on the lives of people who live in this inaccessible "landscape of poverty." Cultivating this imagination requires *not* confusing yourself into thinking that you are able to see life *as* people living in poverty see it, and that you can "imagine the scenery" from their perspective. Hilfiker recommends another version of the balance between what Bakhtin called recognizing each person's nonself-sufficiency—the dependence of each on dialogue with the other—and rejecting the dangerous fantasy of merging consciousness with the other.[20]

Hilfiker's work in the landscape of poverty teaches him that those forced to live there are not noble. He castigates the "myth that the poor are to be our teachers" and finds the idea that poverty teaches virtues to be "attractive fantasies" (186). Those whose lives are forged in poverty are weak—what Levinas calls the face. The more clearly Hilfiker sees this face, the more he fears society's potential to project its darker fantasies onto those who are not noble but are vulnerable: the scapegoating that excludes some people and groups from membership in the community of moral obligation.

Hilfiker recognizes his own urge to scapegoat. Like Campo when he leaves medical school, Hilfiker finds it seductive to blame those whom he is supposed to be helping. Reflection on his own impulses teaches him about society's ungenerous response to those who live in poverty:

I, too, know helpless rage. . . . My self-destructiveness, my indecisiveness, my rage frighten me. They threaten both my sense of self and my chances for success [helping the poor]. It is tempting to protect myself from my own darkness by projecting it onto those poor who suffer on the streets . . . pretending I have nothing in common with Scoop and Bernice, making them wholly "other." (180)

The young Campo makes his patients wholly other by elaborating his checklist of what they are that he is not. Hilfiker, from where he lives and works in the landscape of poverty (if never part of this landscape), recognizes this process happening in society as a whole. We create scapegoats by proving to ourselves that some others lack essential qualities that define who we are. In the current medical milieu, one such defining quality is our individual responsibility to care for our own health. Those who fail on this criterion are thus at fault for their troubles. When scapegoating is extreme, violence is not only acceptable but may be required for the ritual purification of the larger group.[21]

Hilfiker underscores a crucial difference between two ways of dealing with otherness. We can project our self-doubts and rage onto people considered to be other in the sense of the scapegoat: they share so little of what we consider human that we need not honor the commandment not to kill. The opposite way is to value otherness. Valuing otherness begins with Bakhtin's recognition that difference is necessary to sustain dialogue. More relevant to Hilfiker's world is Levinas's responsibility for the face of the other. Hilfiker uses the same metaphor, writing how his and his family's sense of what they were doing in inner-city Washington changed once they began "to see the faces of the poor."[22]

Seeing the face, in all the resonance of that phrase, is essential to avoid the danger of the work Hilfiker does: "Numbness and cynicism, I suspect, are more often the products of frustrated compassion than of evil intentions" (179). Seeing the face is prerequisite to becoming "capable of accepting the world," a phrase that Marcus Aurelius could have said, but is a quotation from Albert Schweitzer.[23] To do the work of poverty medicine, Hilfiker requires a capability to accept a world that includes people making radically different choices for good and bad reasons. That capacity is a requirement for more of human life than practicing poverty medicine.

Hilfiker understands that privileges have made him what he is, and those privileges are part of a pattern that creates the poverty that produces the choices made by his patients. This understanding informs the quotation earlier, in which he underscores the absolute difference between himself and those whose lives have been shaped by poverty. The difference between ways of understanding and acting in the world may seem absolute, yet this difference is part of a single pattern. Within this pattern, Hilfiker finds himself responsible for everyone else, as Levinas says of Dostoevsky's hero.

Hilfiker, like Verghese, Campo, and Alvord, lives in the tension between two worlds. "We [Hilfiker and his wife, Marja] cannot move into the world of the poor," he writes, "but we are no longer quite at home in our own" (115). For Hilfiker as for the others, this external split mirrors an internal separation. He describes himself as "just a human being harboring my own kind of brokenness" (188), implying we all harbor our own brokenness—though few of us have the courage to call it that and to ask what it requires us to do. Those who lack that self-recognition and reflection are prone to project their darker impulses onto others, rendering them scapegoats.

Hilfiker's brokenness provides his dialogical connection with his patients. Early in his book he warns his readers that they may find his religious beliefs alien. As modest as Hilfiker is in referring to his faith, ultimately no other poetic can express his remoralization:

As I stood speaking in the Christ House dining room [a recovery shelter for homeless men, including Hilfiker's patients], I felt almost overwhelmed by the recognition that the pitiable person who stood before me that night in the vestibule and the pitiable person inside me were both children of God. If I could in my own way forgive and even love Scoop [a resident who causes no end of disruption], could I not forgive myself for my own limitations? Could I not allow myself the same love? Not all of us who work with the poor are saints, but maybe we don't have to be. Perhaps sainthood isn't a prerequisite for the job. (188)

Sainthood may not be a prerequisite, but to be a doctor and a human being, Hilfiker must become capable of accepting all the otherness in the world. A prerequisite is to feel responsible for the other's weakness, lest you project your own self-destructiveness onto that other.

Lori Alvord does not use Hilfiker's and Campo's Christian trope of brokenness, but she does recall a childhood in which she felt doubly marginalized. Alvord grew up on reservations, the daughter of a Navajo father and a white mother. She remembers her mother as "loved and accepted" but remaining "slightly outside" Navajo culture. "We learned what it was like to feel peripheral," Alvord writes.[24] She recognizes this feeling as "doubly ironic, because we felt peripheral to a culture that was itself peripheral to the larger culture that engulfed it. We lived on the margin of a margin, which is dangerously close to nowhere at all" (12). This experience of marginality continues when Alvord is recruited to Dartmouth and moves to the world of elite academia: "By my sophomore year I understood what it meant to be invisible. People looked right through me—I moved around the campus as unseen as the air" (28). A third experience of marginality occurs while she is a medical student at Stanford and is hospitalized for a critical infection:

> I noticed things no doctor would ever notice—such as the fact that the hallways were cleaned by large noisy machines in the middle of the night; my roommate would change every few days and another patient and all their relatives would appear, just a curtain away; strangers were constantly coming into my room, unannounced, without introducing themselves, and physically probing my body. Their hands prodded my body. Doctors and nurses gazed into my eyes, and for the first time I was profoundly aware of the experience of a Navajo person in the medical system. (54)[25]

After medical school Alvord practices medicine in the region of New Mexico where she grew up. Unlike Campo, she is able to return to her imaginary homeland. She begins to integrate Navajo emphasis on harmony and balance into her work, trying to perform surgery with an awareness of the "harmony of the entire being" of the patient, and to extend this harmony to relationships among the professionals in the operating room. She takes harmony seriously as a principle of treatment when she attempts to understand a basic surgical problem: why some "successful" operations end with the patient dying.

> From a Navajo standpoint, illness can be caused by an imbalance or lack of harmony in any area of a patient's life. I began to realize that *everything* a patient encounters has an impact on her. If illness could be caused by a lack of harmony, could not the same be true for wellness and the ability to heal? It made sense that if the healing environment was more "harmonious," a patient might return to wellness faster. (74)

Alvord writes that her integration of Navajo beliefs in medical practice, and her participation in traditional healing ceremonies, "helped 'cure' me as well" (101). Here we find her sense of brokenness.

Alvord's commitment to harmony is tested when a little girl, Melanie Begay, is brought to the hospital with clear symptoms of appendicitis. She is accompanied by her Navajo grandmother, Bernice Begay, the family member who would give consent for surgery. Mrs. Begay soon loudly proclaims that "the *bilagáana* doctors were not going to cut open her granddaughter" (139). Alvord admits that the diagnosis for appendicitis is not conclusive; doctors are about 80 percent accurate with female patients, and perhaps less with little girls (139). Those diagnostic odds, together with the low risk involved in the surgery, make the decision obvious, if you believe in Western medicine and the ideas of the body that it depends on. For a Navajo with different beliefs about the body and thus about medicine, it's not at all obvious.

Alvord, conscious of time passing and the risk that a perforated appendix would lead to infection and possibly death, talks to the mother and grandmother, in Navajo as far as she can, and begins to understand their fears. She reflects on the violence that white culture has perpetrated on the Navajo, and the good reasons these women have to be suspicious of white medicine, even when performed by a Navajo doctor. She recalls how frightened she and her sister were when they first entered modern hospitals. "I could see both sides of the story," she writes (143). The medical side sees a high-risk condition that can be treated by low-risk surgery. The Navajo vision sees "the inappropriateness of interfering":

> The beauty of the body would be disturbed. A surgical knife would defile an intact, miniature universe, with rules and systems that evolved naturally over millennia. I could see that sacredness of that body, how all its many parts are one harmonic system. (144)

"The two worlds were colliding" (144), just as two worlds collide when Hilfiker describes patients returning to his clinic after treating their bodies in ways that undermine his earlier efforts to help them; when Campo hears his patient Manuel describing his efforts to become infected with HIV; and when physician readers hear Vanessa Kramer recommending the morality of refusing chemotherapy and radiation.

Alvord chooses to give Mrs. Begay "control of the situation" (145), accepting the risks of delay. Since that risk falls on Melanie, what Alvord accepts is Melanie's place in the local moral experience of her world, as her grandmother represents that experience. In that world, the hypergood is not violating the harmony of the body. The hospital social workers, guided by a different hypergood, were at that moment seeking a court injunction to operate on Melanie. Alvord understands the medical sense of proceeding that way, but she chooses to be guided by her patient's hypergood. Her own Navajo self values this harmony.

Sustaining harmony requires respecting the Begays and the traditions they represent. That respect redefines the risk to Melanie's life, because her life exists only as part of that harmony. Melanie's life has no existence outside the relationships that gave her life and sustain who she uniquely is.

At one point Mrs. Begay seeks Alvord's reassurance that "[y]ou will let us decide the right thing for Melanie" (145), and Alvord says she will. What "the right thing" is, which is always the bioethical question, depends on the prior question of who Melanie is. Is she, as in the Western medical view, an independent physical body that has a right to receive lifesaving treatment? Or is she, as in the Navajo view, a whole that is integral to a larger whole, and that larger whole might be violated if some natural process in her body is disrupted? Alvord's decision, as I understand it, is that Melanie *is* Navajo. She has a right to be treated within those values, with all the risk and benefits (because the two always travel together) that involves.

The story has a happy ending: the family consents to surgery before the appendix perforates. It's clear that Alvord dreads the possibility that Melanie might die, but she accepts that as a risk of respecting the moral world that the little girl is part of. Alvord's writing about ideals of harmony, poetic as it is, can lull us into thinking that something can be achieved without risk. Her story of Melanie reminds us that it can't. Dialogue neither creates nor diminishes risk. It allows us open recognition of all the values that deserve to be considered when responding to the risk that is inherent in being human.

IDENTIFICATION WITH THE ILL

What if Hilfiker's identification with the poor were generalized to physicians identifying with the sick and disabled? As I wrote earlier, Hilfiker does not mean that any of us has to become poor to identify with the poor; on his account, which Levinas would affirm, that sort of identification is impossible. *Identification* begins by recognizing that your landscape is not the other person's. Hilfiker advocates training ourselves to perceive how each personal attitude, each social policy, and each journalistic or academic explanation of behavior will affect those who live in poverty. Identification means constantly asking the question, what will be the material and symbolic effects on them? All Hilfiker claims to have in common with his patients is his brokenness. He lives in an unresolved tension between parts of himself, including parts he can scarcely know. This unalterable otherness within balances his relation to others outside. He cannot know these others, yet he shares a "common community" with them. Identification is the awareness that "each of us is inextricably bound to—indeed, tangled up with—the pain of the poor" (23).

What would it mean for physicians to practice identification with the ill? The dialogical answer is that how the physician conceives of the patient would shift, and part of that shift would be a corresponding change in how physicians imagine themselves. Bakhtin links any understanding of the other with an understanding of the self: "there can be no firm image of the hero answering to the question, 'Who is *he*?' The only questions here are 'Who am *I*' and 'Who are *you*?'" [26] The standard medical response to "Who is he?" is the presentation of patient attributes, beginning with vital signs, moving through diagnosis and treatments, and maybe at the end a "social history" consisting of family status and employment. Bakhtin's radical proposal is that "he" exists only in relation to "I." Who he is depends crucially on who I am, as I address myself to this other.

Bakhtin describes the person as "the subject of an address," which he explains as meaning "One cannot talk about him; one can only address oneself to him" (251). When Bernice Begay, Melanie's grandmother, asks Alvord if she will let the family decide whether to have surgery, she is asking whether Alvord will continue to address herself *to* the family, or whether she will act like a Western doctor and talk *about* the family. The values that mediate Alvord's response to Mrs. Begay—continuing to talk to her, not about her—are as dialogical as they are Navajo.

To identify with the ill, the medical voice needs to speak like a human; that is, to remain in the first and second person. Manuel becomes "you" as he tells Campo his story of years of caring for lovers, loss, and bereavement. The self-destruction inherent in Manuel's behavior does not change, but Campo's willingness to judge Manuel—his compulsion to judge and the distance created by his judgment—shifts. Campo feels a weight shift in his chest, "as though a new passageway were being pried open," as indeed it has. Believing that you have to talk about people, not with them, closes some passageway within us that ought to be open. Identification with the ill is not a burden added to what physicians already bear; it lightens what they must bear.

Since people exist on the boundary with others, who-am-I is always changing in response to who-are-you; our identities can never be stable. Identification with anyone means, paradoxically, recognizing that they are perpetually not identical to what I believed them to be. Bakhtin writes that in Dostoevsky's dialogical novels—these novels being Bakhtin's exemplars, perhaps even his trope, of the moral life—there is "no final, finalizing discourse that defines anything once and forever" (251). No last word can be said about this *you*, whose horizons of possibility remain open. "As long as a person is alive," writes Bakhtin, "he lives by the fact that he is not yet finalized, that he has not yet uttered his ultimate word" (59). Alvord's difficult bioethical decision to delay operating on Melanie respects the unfinalizability of the Begay family, including Melanie. Alvord refuses to usurp the last word that is theirs to utter.

Bakhtin understands the human moral essence as people's acute "sense of their own inner unfinalizability, their capacity to outgrow, as it were, from within and to render *untrue* any externalization and finalizing definition of them" (59). Identification with the ill and disabled respects this "capacity to outgrow," especially when the potential for growth can seem limited, as it appears for Aidan Crane and Jamie Bérubé. Sam Crane and Michael Bérubé claim a distinctly dialogical unfinalizability for their sons. Both Aidan and Jamie have a capacity to outgrow what each now is, but that capacity is more relational than even Bakhtin—who writes of growing "from within"—seems to acknowledge. Aidan, in particular, grows through others' embodied dialogues with him: how they touch him, speak to him, and stimulate his senses. Aidan's and Jamie's "capacity to outgrow" is *from between* themselves and others, not only from within. They are unfinalized as long as others sustain dialogical relationships with them.

The whole comprising unfinalized parts is what Bakhtin calls "The eternal harmony of unmerged voices." He quickly acknowledges, as Marcus would have grumbled he ought to, that these unmerged voices can also be an "unceasing and irreconcilable quarrel" (30). Quarreling, so long as it takes place in dialogue, is a token of each remaining unfinalized for each other. The quarrel turns dangerous when one person finalizes the other, not allowing for change, new beliefs, and new moral images. Then there is no more purpose in talking. Seeking a court order for Melanie Begay's surgery would have ended the dialogue between Alvord and Bernice Begay. It would have finalized them both, and rendered any future harmony not impossible, but far more difficult to attain.

Speaking *to* the other, not *about* him or her, is one way to recognize the unfinalizability of the other. Speaking *about* is not dialogue but monologue, which Bakhtin defines as a condition in which only "one cognitive subject" is allowed, "all else being objects for its cognition" (71, emphases omitted). Alvord, Campo, Hilfiker, and Verghese are taught monological medicine: the doctor is the one cognitive subject in the consulting room, and the patient is object for that cognition. All these physicians discover that this model does not work for them personally—in fact it drives them more or less crazy before they find ways out of it—and it fails their patients. Identification with others requires giving up monologue.

The dialogical end of their respective searches is that each physician reconstitutes him- or herself *in the voices of his or her patients.* When Alvord cedes control of Melanie's surgery to Bernice, she is not only granting her full informed consent. In a dialogical sense, Alvord is allowing the Begay family to be part of who she is as a surgeon. She holds herself open to be reshaped in the voices of future patients; she is as unfinalized as she recognizes them to be. Identification with the ill and disabled thus challenges both medical and commonsense self-understanding of being a self that proceeds outward to meet the world from the standpoint of a stable ego.

Bakhtin reverses our conventional sense (entrenched in our syntax of "I") of there being, in the beginning, a person, a self, who then speaks. Instead, dialogue creates the possibility of becoming a person:

[Dialogue] is not the means for revealing, for bringing to the surface the already ready-made character of a person; no, in dialogue a person not only shows himself outwardly, but he *becomes for the first time* that which he is—and, we repeat, not only for others but for himself as well. To be means to communicate dialogically. When dialogue ends, everything comes to an end. Thus dialogue, by its very essence, cannot and must not come to an end. (252, emphases added)

If that seems too strange a reversal—putting the dialogue before the speakers who "enter" into dialogue—and if it seems impossible to relate to medicine, consider another of the stories Campo tells about what changed him from the person he was to who he became.

If the needle-stick was one epiphany for Campo, another was his

encounter with Aurora, a patient with AIDS. "Aurora was a preopera-
tive male-to-female transsexual according to the terms of some of my
colleagues," he writes; "to others, she was a freak."[27] Campo treats her
more in the freak mode: "I was too busy to notice then the campy
melodrama in her tone of voice; I could barely breathe through my
protective fiberglass-mesh mask [to protect from tuberculosis infec-
tion], and thought only of getting out of her room as soon as possible."
Aurora begins to flirt with Campo; he begins to notice her body and
finds it beautiful. But he remains "too busy to give much thought to
what I had felt" (30). Then she dies.

Campo comes into her room one morning, "expecting her usual
chatter," and finds only silence.

When I rolled her over, seeing her face stripped of all her glittery makeup, expressing not recognition but a deeply subterraneous pain, a primitive and wordless
agony, finally I was moved. As I groped for her, finding her body half-paralyzed
and oddly limp and angular like a bird that has flown into a windowpane, I began
to feel broken myself. I was witnessing the loss of love from the world. Finally in
its absence I was hearing her voice, and when I frantically listened to her heart and
to her lungs for the first and last time I heard the love in them. (32)

Campo writes that when Aurora died later that day,

she left behind an element of herself in me. I find her voice in mine . . . my voice
sounds warmer, more comfortable to me now. I discover her hands on my own
body when I examine a person with cancer, or AIDS. . . . Her glorious eyes return
to me when I finally see someone for the first time. (32)

I read these words not as a merging of voices but as Campo realizing Bakhtin's moral principle that the dialogue "must not come to
an end." Encountering Aurora, Campo "becomes for the first time," in
Bakhtin's phrase. Aurora is dead, but the dialogue she initiated continues in Campo as a person created through this dialogue. Aurora still
speaks through him, not assimilated, but as a new possibility (of compassion, identification, responding to "Who am I?") within Campo. In
this continuing dialogue, Aurora and Campo both remain unfinalized.

Bakhtin describes how a dialogical voice like Campo's, or the other
physicians in this chapter, comes to be:

[H]e receives the word from another's voice and filled with that other voice. The
word enters his context from another context, permeated with the interpretations

of others. His own thought finds the word already inhabited. . . . When there is
no access to one's own personal "ultimate" word, then every thought, feeling, experience must be refracted through the medium of someone else's discourse,
someone else's style, someone else's manner, with which it cannot immediately be
merged without reservation, without distance, with refraction.[28]

That complex passage makes perfect sense when we refract it
through the stories of Campo's encounters with Aurora and Manuel;
of Verghese recognizing what he shares, and what he prays he will
never share, with his patients; of Alvord with the Begays; or of Hilfiker
trying to help patients without requiring them to be who he wants
them to be. All realize that becoming a physician means surrendering
the fantasy of having access to some "ultimate" word and accepting
that their thoughts and voices are refracted through the medium of
their patients' discourse. A complementary refraction takes place for
patients, who must give up their fantasy that the physician can pronounce some ultimate word.

The physician dreams the monological authority of being the single
unquestioned voice. The patient dreams the monological passivity of
having this other pronounce their truth. Healing requires each to give
up his or her respective dream. For the patient, the physician's healing
presence lies in his or her dialogical capacity to take raw and solitary
words of pain and suffering and, dropping the tone of professionalism,
express those words through a human voice, creating something new
between them. For the physician, the patient's healing presence elicits
a new response to the question, "Who am I?" that understands "I"
as coming to be for the first time as the subject of the patient's address, which is the patient's face, his or her weakness. Campo's insight
is that he is as much the subject of Aurora's address as she is the subject of his.

To identify with the other who suffers, in Hilfiker's sense of identification, is not to understand the other. Bakhtin upsets a conventional
humanistic ideal when he observes: "the word 'understanding,' in
its usual, naively realistic interpretation, is always misleading."[29]
Bakhtin, anticipating what Verghese and Hilfiker learn about their relation to their patients, does not believe in "the exact, passive mirroring or duplication of another's experience within myself" (102). He
would affirm Anatole Broyard saying that he does not expect his doctor to suffer with him. So long as "suffering with" is understood as

mirroring or duplication, it's not possible. But a dialogical "suffering with" is possible.

Bakhtin uses suffering as his specific example to propose a different way to comprehend how people understand each other. He begins by reiterating the distance of otherness: "the *other's* suffering as co-experienced by me is in principle different . . . from the other's suffering as *he* experiences it" (102). This distance remains unbridged. But there can develop between us what Bakhtin calls "a completely new *ontic* formation [a thing or being] that I alone actualize *inwardly* from my unique place *outside* another's inner life" (103). Thus there can be "co-experienced suffering" that is not the same as what either person experiences—consciousnesses do not merge—but exists as a new formation that is available, as space of consolation, between self and other.

Bakhtin does not say, nor would his interest be, what the value of this "new ontic formation" might be for the suffering person. This space between offers some outside to the claustrophobia that the self can become. It's a way out of what Campo, describing Aurora's dying face, calls "a primitive and wordless agony." Agony is being locked within, unheard. Going to the space of coexperienced suffering can be consolation. The host whose voice creates this alternative space of co-experienced suffering does not pretend to know what the guest is going through. Rather she or he allows the guest access to the space of what they are going through together, the space that "you," one voice addressed to the other, can create in the tunnel of illness.

What Story Are They Part Of?

We can return to MacIntyre's questions: What story gives these physicians a sense of who they are and what guides them as they wonder what to do?

If one common name were to be given to all four stories in this chapter—and I'm unsure why I feel compelled to make such a conventional gesture of summation, which risks forcing a reconciliation of differences that deserve to remain different—I would call it a diaspora story. The Diaspora was the forced dispersion of the ancient Jews after their Babylonian captivity. Contemporary cultural studies has changed the meaning of *diaspora*, applying the term to the dispersion of many different peoples, under different compulsions. Stuart Hall writes: "diaspora does not refer us to those scattered tribes whose identity can only be secured in relation to some sacred homeland to which they must at all costs return." [30] Instead, diaspora is a metaphor of loss or displacement and of searching for what can never be regained but provides an ideal of what is sought. None of the physician-authors in this chapter is trying to return where they came from: when Verghese searches a map looking for where he might best blend in, he stays within U.S. borders which, for better or worse, have become his horizons. Each realizes that what is of greatest value about that "home" is carried within.

Thus each physician is better described by Hall's definition of the new diaspora:

> The diaspora experience as I intend it here is defined . . . by the recognition of a necessary heterogeneity and diversity; by a conception of "identity" which lives with and through, not despite, difference; by *hybridity*. Diaspora identities are those which are constantly producing and reproducing themselves anew, through transformation and difference. (571)

The story which each physician-author finds him- or herself part of is not an AIDS story, or a Navajo story, or a gay story, or an inner-city story. It's a story of unfinalized hybridity, of unceasing attempts to bring together disparate parts, respecting their otherness (constructing identity, as Hall says, "with and through, not despite, difference"), but believing in a harmony among these parts.

Whether the harmony is known as Alvord's Navajo Beauty Way or Hilfiker's "deep stillness within," [31] it depends on the continuing mutual refraction of selves in words—both words used in traditional ceremonies and words that physicians and patients struggle for, to address each other. Another understanding of the moral moment is when we—two, Bakhtin says, is the minimum—realize that the story is ours to tell: our possibility and our responsibility. But we can tell the story only together, with each other. *We* have to imagine and craft what story *we* find ourselves a part of. That story is the measure of our moral imagination. In a more radical and imperative sense than Broyard intended it, we *all* must make ourselves good stories *for* each other.

CHAPTER FIVE

"So that I can carry on"

*T*HIS chapter tells the story of a palliative care nurse, Linda, and the generosity of the care she offers. Linda, speaking in a brief interview excerpt, describes her relationship with a patient named Miriam Lambert, whose suffering could not be relieved as well as what Linda wants to believe she and her colleagues usually can provide for people who are dying.[2] In contrast to how physicians tell their stories in chapter 4, Linda *speaks* within the immediacy of the work she describes; she does not write, edit, and revise. Her story places

> *[T]he consciousness of the solitary [hero] becomes a field of battle for others' voices; the events of recent days . . . reflected in [her] consciousness, take on the form of a most intense dialogue with absentee participants, and in this dialogue [she] tries to "get [her] thoughts straight."*
> MIKHAIL BAKHTIN[1]
>
> ✻

us, her listeners, in a maelstrom of doubt: Linda doubts how well her attempts to care succeed, and she doubts how generous others' care actually is. Her story evokes the chaos of generosity while it is being practiced, yet she carries on. We can recognize the generosity of her perseverance only when we feel the chaos of her work.

Linda's story is told as one part of an ethnography of Miriam Lambert's final hospitalization and death narrated by Anna Towers, a palliative care physician in Montreal. Several details from Towers's ethnography set the context for Linda's story. Mrs. Lambert was sixty-eight when she was admitted to the palliative care unit of the hospital shortly after having been diagnosed as having melanoma that had spread from her foot to her pelvis and spine. Her partner, whom she had never married, was a ninety-eight-year-old man who had moved to a nursing home six months before her diagnosis; they had no children. In one interview she describes herself by saying, "I don't know who I am" (179). At the time of diagnosis she says to her brother: "How can my life be ending? It hasn't started yet" (181).

Mrs. Lambert is admitted to the palliative care unit because of her uncontrollable pain. Towers explains the clinical problem: "When pain is due to tumor invasion of nerves, opioids alone are not sufficient to control it" (181). Much of Mrs. Lambert's case history describes different attempts at pain control, and the chapter concludes with a "medication and pain control record" detailing drugs, dosages, and other pain-relief interventions (192–95). Just as Linda wants to assure herself that she did everything she could for Mrs. Lambert, so the book's authors want to convince the reader that all possible pain medications were tried. For Mrs. Lambert, however, none worked.

Complete remission of pain, however fortunate when it is achieved, is not the preeminent clinical objective in palliative care, since increased medication doses have side-effects that include decreased lucidity. The preferred treatment is to alter the patient's experience of pain so that less medication is necessary. Towers writes that in other end-of-life cases "the pain would still be there, but it would be experienced differently, and the suffering reduced. The patient would reach a deeper level of understanding, almost as if the suffering had been given new meaning" (189). Towers thus summarizes palliative care's preferred story: care is supposed to facilitate "a deeper level of understanding" that has physical effects including reduced need for pain medication. Yet the collective opinion of those caring for Mrs. Lambert is that she never experiences this transformation. Maybe the physical source of her pain rendered it intractable. Doubt remains what else could have been done. Mrs. Lambert is admitted to palliative care on August 30, 1996, and she dies on December 5.

Linda is the pseudonym that Towers gives to one of Mrs. Lambert's primary care nurses. Around November 25, Linda sought out Anna Towers, to talk about caring for Mrs. Lambert. Calling the context of Linda's storytelling an interview reduces the multiple involvements of Linda and Anna Towers in their dialogue. Towers plays several roles: Linda's (unquoted) interlocutor, a consulting physician on Mrs. Lambert's case, and a researcher, in which capacity she recorded their conversation. We do not know how much she is also Linda's friend. As Linda tells her story, she seems to be speaking from within different relationships to her listener. These multiple relationships mean that

Linda must speak in different voices, as different parts of her story are addressed to someone who embodies different listeners all at once. "All at once" is a key phrase Linda uses to describe the chaos of her work. The shifting voices of her story mirror her work's multiple demands and overlapping relationships.

Linda's story—part confession, part case report, part critique— seems to pour out of her. She seems to be hearing herself say these un- controllable words and as she listens—and sees what we cannot see, her words' effect on her partner in dialogue—she weighs the implica- tions of what she says. The authors of *Crossing Over* render Linda's story in syntactically correct prose before their readers see it. I have tamed the story further by inserting additional paragraph indenta- tions. Even edited in these ways, Linda's story retains the jagged edges of its telling. Linda sometimes speaks of herself in the third person; she employs a variety of verb tenses (suggesting at one point that Mrs. Lambert has already died); pronouns near the end of the story have unclear referents; and the narrative moves between at least two different physical places, with minimal marking of transition between these spaces.

Linda not only describes a chaotic situation, she evokes the chaos. As we read the story in neat sentences and paragraphs, it's hard to imagine how fresh and raw it must have been as Linda spoke it.

I'd like to speak now, because after they die, I forget. That's how I protect myself, I guess. I'm remembering everything that she said now, but when they die, I for- get. I have to forget so that I can carry on with the next patient.

In the beginning, her pain was uncontrollable. One day she had severe electric shock-like pains that made her scream. She knew that her screaming wouldn't up- set me and that knowledge reassured her. She appreciated getting consistent nursing care. She leaned on her two primary nurses quite heavily.

I entered her pain at one point. I was in pain, too. We had tried absolutely everything and nothing was working. On that day, my neck went into spasm from stress and I had to go home early because of the pain. I had had neck pain in the past, but when I feel that people need me all at once, my neck pain comes back. I knew then that I had overstepped my boundary and that I couldn't get so involved.

She greeted me crying, saying she'd never get out of bed again because of the pain, and she never did. She told me that her emotional pain is more than her physical pain.

She has learned to express her needs, which she had difficulty doing before. She is able to ask volunteers for help. She makes volunteers feel special.

However, she realized that some people may come for their own comfort and not hers.

Sometimes we need to feel that we are doing something, but it doesn't help. (190–91)

PALLIATIVE CARE AS POLYPHONY

Linda's story reflects a tension between palliative care's commitment to dialogue and the monologue that characterizes most medical narration. Bakhtin's statement of how Dostoevsky's dialogical writing disrupts the monological novel could be describing both Towers's ethnography and Linda's style of narration:

Indeed, the monological unity of the world is destroyed in a Dostoevskian novel, but those ripped-off pieces of reality are in no sense directly combined in the unity of the novel: each of these pieces gravitates toward the integral field of vision of a specific character; each makes sense only at the level of a specific consciousness.[3]

Medical case reports—charts and presentations in rounds—aspire to monological unity. The speaking or writing voice denies that the reality it expresses "makes sense only at the level of a specific consciousness." Other, lesser voices speak from their particular perspectives. The monological voice speaks from beyond such limitation, and thus claims authority. Monologue silences other voices. Dialogue, on the other hand, invites response, because each dialogical voice recognizes its own limitation.

In contrast with the monological medical style, Towers's entire ethnography reads like Bakhtin's "ripped-off pieces of reality" that converge in dialogue. Linda's narration is one of those pieces, and it in turn comprises other ripped-off pieces: other stories that could be told in other voices. Principal among these is Mrs. Lambert's voice, which Linda both quotes and paraphrases; then the voices of Mrs. Lambert's family and of medical staff and volunteers who cared for her; and beyond all these we can hear voices of social expectations, fears, and hopes about dying. It's crucial to dialogue that only in a couple of sentences near the end of her story does Linda assimilate Mrs. Lambert's voice to her own, in order to speak *about* her.

A dialogical response to Linda's story is to refrain from putting these ripped-off pieces together, which would manufacture the illusory integration of monologue that Linda struggles to carry on without. Conventional usage suggests the phrase "putting them *back* together." But for the Dialogical Stoic, there is no original unity to be regained; that unity is a monological fantasy. This chapter's epigraph with Bakhtin's metaphor of "a field of battle for others' voices" describes both Linda's method of narration and the context of her narrative. Linda recognizes Bakhtin's dialogical principle: that each piece of her story makes sense only at the level of her specific consciousness. Yet her consciousness is a *polyphony* of voices, to use Bakhtin's preferred term. Linda struggles to live with the unmerged voices that swirl in her head, each piece competing to describe both what palliative care ought to be, and what Linda ought to be in relation to her patients and colleagues. In polyphony the competing voices create a harmony that never unifies them but holds them in mutual dependence. The voices are parts of a whole in which they remain distinct but are interdependent.

This harmony can be hard to hear—Linda's doubts come at the end of her story—but generosity requires belief in harmony. *Chaos* is voices in competition with no harmony. This chaos is an ever-present danger of Linda's work. One of Linda's tasks, as she attempts to "get her thoughts straight" about her patient, her work, herself, and the possibility of generosity in care of the dying, is to reassure herself that there *is* a harmony among the polyphonic voices. At the end of her story, the harmony is not assured—it will never be assured. Yet Linda seems to have regained the perseverance she needs to "carry on."

Linda's way of being a nurse is a hands-on practice of what Bakhtin describes as authorship of a polyphonic novel. What he says of the author also describes the good nurse:

The author of a polyphonic novel is not required to renounce himself or his own consciousness, but he must to an extraordinary extent broaden, deepen and rearrange this consciousness . . . in order to accommodate the autonomous consciousnesses of others. This was a very difficult and unprecedented project . . . [but] it was essential if the polyphonic nature of life itself was to be artistically recreated. (68)

Linda approaches each of her patients with an expectation that she will be called to "broaden, deepen, and rearrange" her consciousness, "in order to accommodate the autonomous consciousness" of that patient.

Palliative care is committed to *polyphonic caring:* it aspires to accommodate autonomous voices rather than assimilate them into its own preferred monologue.[4] Palliative care is distinguished not by its expertise in pain control, crucially important as this skill is, or by caring for patients whose death is anticipated to be imminent. What truly distinguishes it is that it resists the impulse to unify and finalize what can be said about patients within the single voice of scientific knowledge and technological control. Instead, palliative care is dialogical: it seeks to expand not only what patients say about themselves but also the capacity of caregivers to hear what their patients say.

Linda remains a medical professional—medicine is one voice she must accommodate. But she is a palliative care worker in her unrelenting attempt to honor what Bakhtin calls "the polyphonic nature of life," with its multiple autonomous consciousnesses. Her story presents no single, monological field of vision, but "several fields of vision, each full and of equal worth."[5] Linda's constant risk of chaos is that those several fields will conflict in the incompatible demands they assert. In caring for Mrs. Lambert, the polyphony turns to chaos.

LINDA'S BOUNDARY

The climax of Linda's story seems to be when she "enters" Mrs. Lambert's pain. She describes her neck spasms as the result of having "overstepped my boundary." This description recalls Bakhtin's statement that is the epigraph of chapter 2: "A person has no internal sovereignty, he is wholly and always on the boundary; looking inside of himself, he looks into the eyes of another or with the eyes of another" (287). Being in dialogue with the other person is to be on this boundary. Being on the boundary is unstable: overstepping in either direction is a danger, but life presents no choice. For Bakhtin, dialogue is what prevents "absolute death," which he defines as "the state of being unheard, unrecognized, unremembered" (287). Palliative care accepts that bodies will die, and that's no embarrassment, as Marcus reminds himself. But palliative care seeks to prevent the absolute death—being unheard, unrecognized, unremembered. It is this death, not the death of the body, that offends the human dignity of both dying persons and those who care for them.

While Linda attempts to prevent Mrs. Lambert's "absolute death," she oversteps her boundary. Linda attempts to hear Mrs. Lambert, but Mrs. Lambert seems unable to recognize herself as one capable of being heard. As Linda reaches over the boundary toward her patient, she literally feels with Mrs. Lambert's muscles. Her own muscles go into spasm. This doesn't help, to quote the last line in her story. Linda has "to go home early because of the pain." *Early* here seems to mean more than before her shift ends. Linda goes home prematurely, before Mrs. Lambert can be heard. Linda's work is to remain present in order to hear, but her muscle spasms interrupt that work. Linda does not describe her return to the unit; we as her listeners are confronted, as suddenly as she must have felt she was, by Mrs. Lambert's outpouring of tears and words. I sensed that Mrs. Lambert had to contain these until Linda's return allowed their release. What Mrs. Lambert then says about herself will be discussed shortly. For now the focus is on Linda, boundaries, and dialogue.

Linda places herself on the boundary between herself and her patients. She practices, every day in her work, the balance described in chapter 2 between what Bakhtin calls "nonself-sufficiency," which people have to recognize to remain human, and the danger of merging in the consciousness of the other. Literary critic Tzvetan Todorov describes this balance by suggesting "three kinds of human relations." As is often the case in Bakhtinian studies, what Todorov writes about the critic's relation to an author can be read as a physician's or nurse's relation to a patient.

The first [human relation] consists in unifying in the name of the self: the critic projects himself in the work he reads, and all authors illustrate or exemplify his thought. The second kind corresponds to the "criticism of identification".... The critic has no proper identity, there is but one identity, that of the author under examination, and the critic becomes his; we witness a kind of ecstatic fusion, and therefore once again we have unification. The third kind would be the dialogue advocated by Bakhtin, where each of the two identities remains affirmed (there is neither integration nor identification), where knowledge takes the form of a dialogue with a "thou" equal to the "I" and yet different from it. As with creation, Bakhtin gives empathy, or identification, merely a preparative, transitory role.[6]

In the first kind of relationship—"unifying in the name of the self"—the clinician-patient relationship is all about medicine. The second relationship—ecstatic fusion—is a surfeit of empathy: it's all about the patient, but not in a way that helps. Both are monologues: either assimilating the other to oneself, or fusing oneself with the other. In the third relationship, it's about the dialogue between them. Empathy, however that slippery word is specified, is necessary as preparation for dialogue; unifying in the name of the self has no empathy, and it doesn't help. But when empathy becomes ecstatic fusion, this boundary crossing forestalls dialogue.

Linda's muscle spasm is the ecstatic fusion that Todorov refers to: a caring relationship of identification or, more accurately, unification. Linda's commitment to the philosophy of palliative care predisposes her to this extreme, since palliative care is founded in the attempt to avoid the medical analogue of Todorov's first kind of literary criticism: using the patient to illustrate or exemplify medical skill at diagnosis and intervention.[7] Linda seems to feel pulled to the extreme of identification by the difficulty of engaging Mrs. Lambert in a dialogue that ought to take place in a space between them. If dialogue were situated between nurse and patient, Linda could enter it and still remain who she is, on her side of that space.

This dialogical space between can only exist if both enter together; yet not everyone is prepared to enter dialogue, for all sorts of reasons. Mrs. Lambert's statement quoted earlier, that her life "hasn't started yet," suggests that she has not yet begun to enter dialogical relationships. On Bakhtin's account, life begins in dialogue; Linda's appraisal confirms this interpretation. Elsewhere in the ethnography of Mrs. Lambert's care, Towers quotes Linda saying, "I couldn't get down in there, like I can with other patients."[8] Bakhtin might encourage Linda to imagine getting *between* there—getting into the boundary space between herself and her patients—rather than *down* there, a metaphor that precipitates the risk of sinking into the patient and overstepping the boundary.

Bakhtin would also recognize the danger that is precipitated when the absence of dialogue is described as the result of something lacking in Mrs. Lambert. It becomes easy to imagine "incapable of dialogue" written in some patient's chart, designating a failure of capacity or will. Such undialogical words would finalize Mrs. Lambert and thus be a form of violence against her. Linda's clinical problem is to stop well short of such diagnostic finalization of Mrs. Lambert, but be able to imagine that this patient is unprepared, for all sorts of reasons, to enter the dialogue her palliative care hosts hope to engage her in. This imagination can, paradoxically, keep dialogue open because it helps

Linda to avoid overstepping the boundary and the resulting foreclosure of dialogue.

Linda's experience caring for Mrs. Lambert seems to confirm Bakhtin's insistence that we live on the boundary with others, but it underscores the danger of that relationship. It can be difficult to keep your balance on a boundary. If the other person does not balance our presence on our side of the boundary with his or her presence on the other side, then we fall either back into ourselves or forward into the other. To fall back is to see others as exemplifying our thoughts about them and purposes for them. To fall forward risks ecstatic fusion.

Does Linda overstep her boundary, or does Mrs. Lambert, who has little experience of dialogue, pull Linda over, making fusion the only possibility? This question can never be resolved; it's one of the doubts that Linda has to live with. And it raises another question that is even more troubling: does Mrs. Lambert's dignity require that she be allowed to die as she has lived, even if that death is, by her own report and others' observation, an unhappy one? When does generosity indicate staying not only on your own side of the boundary, but even a bit back from it, lest you infringe on the other's side and violate what makes them *other*? We thus come to a concept at the core of Levinas's thought: alterity.

ALTERITY

Todorov posits two forms of monological relationships—projecting onto and merging with—and a third, preferred form, which is dialogue. The basis of dialogue is a relationship of otherness: sufficient difference and distance so that there can be a space between two people. Mrs. Lambert's otherness seems unlike that described in previous stories. In stories of Verghese's and Campo's AIDS patients, Hilfiker's inner-city patients, and Alvord's Navajo patients, otherness implies being marginal to the mainstream of society (the postulation of a mainstream being necessary for some people to be considered marginal). Otherness also implies one person's alienation from others as a result of differences in social situation. This alienation is at least diminished, if never entirely overcome, through dialogue. Campo is alienated from Manuel's self-destructive desire to contract AIDS. He feels estranged from a patient who seems less a fellow human being because of the inhuman choices he makes. But as Campo listens, Manuel's otherness appears as a tragic contingency of different personal histories. Campo still does not approve of Manuel's choices—he would, if he could, persuade him to act differently—but the sense of being with a fellow human is restored.

Otherness in Campo's story seems to depend on attributes, whether these are differences of being healthy or sick, differences of sexual orientation, differences that derive from being situated in a minority culture, or differences of access to privilege. Thinking about Linda's difficulty of engaging Mrs. Lambert in dialogue requires a concept of otherness that transcends—or precedes—such attributes.

Levinas calls this noncontingent otherness *alterity,* from the Latin *alter,* "other." The jargon is justified, because Levinas needs a new word if he is to describe a difference that precedes what are generally thought of as differences. Alterity does not depend on the contingency of when and where someone is born or what life choices he or she makes. Alterity is an intrinsic quality of being human; for Levinas, it may be *the* intrinsic human quality. Moreover, it *precedes* such specific differences as gender, age, ethnicity, or state of health. Levinas writes:

It is not because your hair is unlike mine or because you occupy another place than me—this would only be a difference of properties or of dispositions in space, a difference of attributes. But before any attribute, you are other than I, other otherwise, absolutely other! And it is this alterity, different from the one which is linked to attributes, that is your alterity.[9]

Levinas makes respect for alterity one of his core moral imperatives. Just as Bakhtin believes one person must not pronounce final words about another, Levinas believes that to infringe on the other person's alterity—their otherness that precedes any attributes—is to commit violence against the other. Symbolic violence comprises the often subtle ways that alterity is challenged and violated. This violence claims to object to specific choices and decisions, but the objection shifts from the choice to the person choosing. It's the violence of telling people that they should not be who they are, or that they fail to understand who they ought to be.

The most pernicious symbolic violence tells people that their personal and cultural history, which underlies their hypergoods, is wrong. It would have been symbolically violent for Lori Alvord to have told Bernice Begay that she was absolutely, culpably wrong to deny surgery for her granddaughter. Alvord, as a physician, should disagree with Mrs. Begay, but her form of disagreement—making her case in favor of surgery and then leaving the final decision to the Begay family—is a model of dialogue that honors alterity. Alvord does not tell the Begays they have to be anyone other than who they are. But she also stays with them; she does not leave them to suffer alone.

Medicine, therapeutic work generally, and education are especially at risk of committing symbolic violence, because professionals in these fields speak with an authority deriving from both their expertise and their claim to be acting in the client's best interest. People come to doctors, nurses, therapists, and teachers because they want something changed: they want their illness cured, or they want their lives to improve, or they want to learn something they do not yet know. People—as patients, clients, and students—want authority. It thus becomes all too easy for professionals to forget that people also want to be respected for who they already are. The professional finds it too easy to see the client's need or lack, move to some solution or remedy for that, and miss the face.

Levinas's ethic begins with seeing the *face* of the other—the other's vulnerability and weakness, as described in chapter 2. Seeing the face often begins with the empathic imagination of how the other feels, but empathy risks the symbolic violence of telling the other how to feel better. Alterity is not opposed to empathy (or to feeling better), but empathy as an end in itself can be dangerous to alterity. Empathy tends toward unification: either my projecting what would make me feel better onto you, or my fusing with your suffering. Alterity is the opposite of unification with the other.[10] Seeing the face requires respect for alterity: I must recognize that there are aspects of your suffering that I can never imagine and that I can never touch.

Alterity is the dynamic that drives the dialogical relationship. It is the difference that makes dialogue possible, and one goal of dialogue is to sustain alterity. The first two forms of human relationship described above by Todorov—assimilation of the other into my voice, or submerging myself in the other—terminate dialogue by violating alterity. When Linda, for the most generous of motives, oversteps the boundary between herself and Mrs. Lambert, she violates Mrs. Lambert's alterity, and dialogue breaks down. The hard truth of Mrs. Lambert's care is that Linda can best recognize her patient's face by staying *with* her—never abandoning her, yet *apart* from her; not merging with her.

Bakhtin writes: "Everything in [Dostoevsky's] world lives on the very border of its opposite."[11] He might have added that everything can remain alive only so long as it lives on that border. The border requires, on each side, something different from what is on the other side; to assimilate the other or to merge oneself into the other is to lose the opposition. Alterity sustains dialogue, and thus life. But alterity is also what makes dialogue difficult, simply because the other *is* other. For Linda, alterity is painful, even before her neck goes into spasm. But overstepping the boundary ends dialogue. It shifts the pain to her body, but it doesn't help.

What, then, is Mrs. Lambert's alterity? She speaks of her "emotional pain," the pain that exceeds any physical suffering. Linda describes Mrs. Lambert's pain as what makes it difficult for this patient to express her needs. This emotional pain sets Mrs. Lambert apart, because she *is* apart, and so the cycle continues. But the "what is alterity?" question, with its demand for specification and explanation, risks symbolic violence. Alterity is not a container of specific attributes, whether psychological, cultural, or physical, that can be taken out and examined. To specify any person's alterity is to seek to finalize it. To specify Mrs. Lambert's alterity is to assimilate her into a unifying voice that claims to explain her. In the unity of that explanation, there is no space for unexplained difference; so alterity evaporates, explained away.

Alterity is not ineffable—it's not that of which it is impossible to speak—but violence is risked when too much is spoken. Specification turns into the symbolic violence of finalizing the other when it reduces this person to some set of inherent properties that explain why he or she is a problem, and why that problem could not be solved.

One aspect of Linda's generosity is her refusal to diagnose Mrs. Lambert as being a difficult patient; that would be symbolic violence. Toward the end of Linda's story she describes Mrs. Lambert in a third-person, clinical voice of speaking about: "She has learned . . . She is able . . . She makes . . . " But then, as I will discuss in the next section, Linda allows alterity to return when she sees the clinic through Mrs. Lambert's eyes: "she realized . . . " Her interrogation of who Mrs. Lambert is turns into Mrs. Lambert's assessment of who Linda and her colleagues are. Linda's generosity is her realization that who-you-are depends on who-I-am. Both identities are processes and questions, and these questions can only be posed in reciprocity.

CHAOS AND DOUBT

Linda has had neck pain in the past, she says. The pain comes back "when I feel that people need me all at once." The chaos that challenges Linda's generosity seems crystallized in that "all at once." In these overlapping and perhaps conflicting demands, not only Linda's consciousness but also her time and bodily involvement are "a field of battle," as Bakhtin writes in this chapter's epigraph. The polyphony loses its harmony and begins to sound like a cacophony. Chaos results when Linda can no longer "get her thoughts straight."

The chaos of sheer demand is compounded by doubt. In the first half of Linda's story she doubts herself; her overstepping her boundary marks a limit of her ability to help Mrs. Lambert. In the second half of her story, the doubt spreads outward: Linda doubts the motives of her colleagues, and she may doubt palliative care itself.

Linda's expressions of doubt begin after she describes Mrs. Lambert telling her about her emotional pain. At this point in her story Linda changes tone. "Emotional pain" labels the distance between Mrs. Lambert and those who care for her, but the label does not reduce this distance. The phrase marks Linda's inability to use dialogue to shift the intensity of Mrs. Lambert's physical pain through that dialogue. Faced with this inability to talk *with* Mrs. Lambert, Linda begins to talk *about* her. Linda speaks in what can be called chart talk. She assesses Mrs. Lambert in the style of a clinical report card: "She has learned to express her needs, which she had difficulty doing before. She is able to ask volunteers for help. She makes volunteers feel special." In these sentences, Mrs. Lambert is no longer a dialogical partner whose consciousness is respected in its alterity. She is someone who has, to whatever degree, met institutional expectations. She is assessed as having gotten right the task of being a patient. Linda assesses her, on balance, as a good patient. That assessment is professional monologue.

Dialogue returns as Linda's talk shifts from an assessment of Mrs. Lambert to Mrs. Lambert's own assessment of the palliative care unit. Linda's voice merges with Mrs. Lambert's voice, and the doubt about the motives of "some people" seems to be theirs jointly. This assessment cuts to the core of clinical generosity: "she realized that some people may come for their own comfort and not hers." It's not clear who "some people" are. The syntax suggests the earlier referent, volunteers, but Linda's storytelling does not follow strict syntactic rules. Linda's last sentence expands who may be included in those who come for their own comfort, not for the patient. "Sometimes we need to feel that we are doing something, but it doesn't help," Linda says. "We" now seems to include Linda herself and all her colleagues. Doubt spreads through all of palliative care.

Linda's doubts, echoing Mrs. Lambert's and extending what she may have said, are endemic to generosity. The cultural historian Jean Starobinski concludes his history of gift giving as depicted in art and poetry by observing that generosity always elicits doubt. What Starobinski calls the "simulacra" of gifts can be understood either as counterfeit gifts or as real gifts given for counterfeit motives.

Have people not always divined and denounced the countless simulacra that accompany the gift like its own shadow, thus eliciting doubt about the generosity of intentions, the legitimacy of dispersed riches, the quality of the metal in the coins distributed? Have we not seen, in every era, charlatans who made people believe that overabundance sprang directly from them as they threw out handfuls of inferior products? . . . It is the serpent who sometimes whispers in our ear that the gifts we are witnessing are not true gifts, but only the guise of egoism.[12]

We cannot know what Mrs. Lambert sees or hears that leads to her judgment. Some of the care offered her may well be "only the guise of egoism." Or, we can recall Bakhtin's description (in chapter 2) of how the human consciousness of self is formed: "I realize myself initially through others: from them I receive words, forms, and tonalities for the formation of my initial idea of myself." Bakhtin goes on to say that we remain affected by "the elements of infantilism in self-awareness," including the question of who can love a person like me. These questions are more serpents that whisper in our ears, sometimes "until the end of life."[13]

The intractable chicken-and-egg dilemma of Mrs. Lambert's doubts about the generosity of her care is whether some "element of infantilism" in her self-awareness prevents her from accepting the consolation that others offer. Mrs. Lambert may project her inability to feel loved onto others. She may then believe that they cannot love her, and that they care for her only for their own sake, not hers. But an alternative is equally plausible. Perhaps Mrs. Lambert, who is not afraid of being alone, has the courage to recognize and express what other patients find it more comfortable to ignore or remain silent about: some people do "come for their own comfort." This recognition requires courage because it denies Mrs. Lambert some of the consolation that she might take from others.

However Mrs. Lambert's doubts are motivated, and whatever she recognizes or misrecognizes, her doubts elicit and seem to complement Linda's own doubts, as expressed in Linda's closing pronouncement. One interpretation of the last sentence is that Linda is completing a confessional apology for overstepping her boundary and having had to go home, abandoning Mrs. Lambert. Linda's neck spasm is a way she was able to feel she was doing something—if she cannot relieve Mrs. Lambert's pain, she can at least identify with this pain so closely that she goes into spasm. But Linda realizes this doesn't help Mrs. Lambert. Her neck spasm crosses a boundary between empathy and egoism: it's about the caregiver feeling how much she is doing, and it ends dialogue. In palliative care, an end to talk is inevitable; the prognosis of imminent death is the criterion for patient admission. This end to talk need not end dialogue; it need not leave Mrs. Lambert unheard.

At one point in Linda's story, a listener could readily forget that Mrs. Lambert is still alive. Linda comments about Mrs. Lambert's prediction that she would never get out of bed: "and she never did" (not "she never has"), a choice of tense implying that Mrs. Lambert has died. As Linda says at the start of her story, she is remembering Mrs. Lambert in preparation for her death, when Linda says she will forget. Before then, in an act of generosity, Linda carries on this intense dialogue with a participant who seems simultaneously present and absent. Unlike Barry Siegler, the physician described in chapter 1, Linda willingly opens a Pandora's box full of doubt about her own capacity to care, and doubts about her colleagues. She lapses into a few sentences of speaking about Mrs. Lambert, but then allows Mrs. Lambert's voice to speak through her. She never dismisses Mrs. Lambert as a patient who has "failed" palliative care, as Vanessa Kramer's cancer center dismisses her as having "failed" her treatment protocol. Linda sustains a dialogue with Mrs. Lambert, and in that dialogue, Mrs. Lambert is, most definitely, not dead.

STILL LEARNING FROM MRS. LAMBERT

What makes Linda a good nurse, in the moral sense of good, and how does her telling of her story renew generosity in medicine? Why not retell some of palliative care's good-death stories, in which the caring environment transforms suffering? Do not those stories better present the remoralization of medicine?

My reasons for choosing Mrs. Lambert's story begin with Linda's initial comment that she needs to "carry on." Stoics carry on; they're soldiers, used to being in the muck and fray. Linda's storytelling performs a Stoic exercise of sorting out the internal—whatever affects her character and is her responsibility—from the external, which cannot harm her. What did she allow herself to perceive, and how did she act on the perceptions she chose to acknowledge? The external includes the contingency of Mrs. Lambert's disease and the difficulty of pain control that disease creates. Linda says that she was not upset by Mrs. Lambert's screaming in pain. Like a well-trained Stoic, Linda chooses how to interpret the screaming and how to respond to it. Her calm "reassured" Mrs. Lambert.

What is internal, and where she does less well in her own estimation, includes Linda's overstepping her boundary. Also internal are Linda's doubts, through which she must carry on. I think that on most days Linda would agree with Starobinski, who concludes his discussion of generosity's shadow with a rhetorical question that reaffirms generosity: "But who could deny that, in the face of enormous distress, the need to give is still very much alive or that institutions do devote themselves to giving with true compassion?"[14] Linda does not doubt the compassion she and her colleagues give to Mrs. Lambert. Sharing doubts with, and about, Mrs. Lambert is part of Linda's continuing dialogue with her. Linda works every day "in the face of enormous distress." She faces not only the chaos of everyone needing her at once, but also the chaos of doubt about her own and others' compassion. She carries on.

Linda's generosity is described by one of Bakhtin's contemporary critics of Russian literature, whom he quotes with approval:

[Russian criticism of Dostoevsky] is still learning from Ivan Karamazov and Rashkalnikov . . . entangling itself in the same contradictions that entangled them, stopping in bewilderment before the problems that they failed to solve and bowing respectfully before their complex and tormenting experience.[15]

Linda is still learning from Mrs. Lambert. Perhaps Linda will forget details of Mrs. Lambert's care as she carries on with her next patient. But her storytelling keeps her entangled in the contradictions of Mrs. Lambert's life and death. Linda stops in bewilderment before puzzles that the palliative care team will never solve—what comes first: Mrs. Lambert's difficulty in accepting relationships of care, or the element of egoism in how some people offer care? She ultimately bows respectfully before an experience as tormenting as Dostoevsky could have imagined. She becomes a hero in Bakhtin's sense of one who sustains dialogue.

Linda's care of Mrs. Lambert exemplifies the moral relationship according to Levinas:

"Thou shalt not kill" is also the fact that I cannot let the other die alone. There is, as it were, an appeal to me. You see . . . the relation with the other is not symmetrical.[16]

When you have encountered a human being, you cannot simply leave him alone. Most of the time one leaves things; one says, "I've done everything!" But that is just it—no, one has done nothing! (216)

Linda is the good nurse who cannot leave the other to die alone, who enters the asymmetry of the relation with Mrs. Lambert, and who resigns herself to the paradox that when she has done everything, not enough has been done. Linda cannot leave Mrs. Lambert alone, in the sense of solitary, but she learns to leave her alone, in the sense of respecting her alterity. Respecting alterity sustains the boundary between them, and the boundary sustains dialogue.

Not leaving Mrs. Lambert to die alone includes not only being present at her bedside but also letting Mrs. Lambert's voice speak, no matter how much Linda herself is destabilized, rendered out of control, by the voice that she cannot get "down in there" with. Mrs. Lambert's alterity tests Linda's generosity. Linda could use psychosocial assessment language to drown out this voice whose otherness is threatening, but she doesn't. I choose her story because it is on the boundary of chaos: the chaos of screaming, of muscles in spasm, of emotional pain, of doubting why some people are there, and questioning what is done for the sake of seeming to do something, even though it doesn't help. Amid this chaos of tormenting experience, Linda carries on. Hers is a generosity before which we can bow respectfully.

CHAPTER SIX

Unfinalized Generosity

A SCENE of modern generosity—showing both its gains and what has been given up for those gains—is depicted by Michael Ignatieff, writing about social welfare. Ignatieff describes his relationships with the elderly, "respectably poor" people who are his neighbors in London. Or at least he and they live in the same neighborhood. The extent to which they can be each other's moral neighbor is the question.

Must one despair of seeing the triumph of the pure gift, the gift without compensation, the gift given without consideration for one's own interest? Would it not be preferable to return to the Stoic god by giving . . . without striking a bargain where those who worked to relieve human suffering would be remunerated with future happiness?

JEAN STAROBINSKI

As we stand together in line at the post office, while they cash their pension cheques, some tiny portion of my income is transferred into their pockets through numberless capillaries of the state. The mediated quality of our relationship seems necessary to both of us. They are dependent on the state, not upon me, and we are both glad of it. Yet I am also aware of how this mediation walls us off from each other. We are responsible for each other, but we are not responsible to each other.[1]

Ignatieff is responsible for his neighbors, insofar as he pays his small fraction of their pensions. But not responsible to them; he need not see their faces.

The line at the post office reminds me of waiting rooms in medical clinics. In the Canadian clinics where I am a patient, some of us are paying more, in taxes, to sit in the same waiting room with others who pay less. I feel fortunate to live in a country that extends the language of rights to medical treatment.[2] Yet I recognize that defining a service as a right removes it from the sphere of generosity. This shift of spheres is a gain both of certainty and of equality. The pensioners who stand beside Ignatieff in the post office can depend on their checks arriving on time, and they can greet Ignatieff as equals, not as those beholden to a benefactor. Those who sit next to me in waiting rooms in Canadian clinics can feel confident that ability to pay will not affect their access to a physician—though their access to prescription medicines is less assured. They know that if they need surgery or other critical care, they will not have to mortgage their homes—though how long they may have to wait can be a problem. These advantages are so transparently clear that we can forget what has been lost.

Ignatieff sees the loss clearly: giver and recipient become walled off from each other by layers of mediation and regulation. In the clinic, physicians and nurses are hardly postal clerks who dole out services that have been allocated elsewhere. But the physician-patient relationship is mediated, whether that mediation is by government as the single-payer, as in the Canadian and other publicly funded systems, or by some private insurer, as in the United States. Generosity is constrained by regulation, or people *feel* constrained, which produces the same effect.

How did we get to this modern form of mediated generosity? In 1990 the Louvre mounted an exhibition of artworks that reveal cultural imaginations of gift giving, especially acts of charity, from the ancient world to the present. The guest curator, critic and cultural historian Jean Starobinski, wrote an accompanying monograph that is the most complete cultural history of generosity as charity. Starobinski suggests three historical periods of generosity: ancient, Christian, and Enlightenment.

Starobinski's description of gift giving among the ancient Romans anticipates Levinas's emphasis on the nonreciprocity of generosity: "The act of giving without being paid in return placed a man almost among the ranks of the divine." He quotes several ancient writers on the theme that a person's spiritual possessions cannot exceed what they have given away as material gifts. "Only the god of the Stoics could give without expecting anything in return," Starobinski concludes; "that expectation would have been a lack incompatible with divine perfection."[3]

Yet the generosity of the ancients does not seem dialogical. The Stoic gives from within the inner citadel of the self, the gift seeming more a token of the giver's moral competence, his or her character, than a boundary point at which two meet. The gift is not the token of the mutual effect that giver and receiver have on each other within a dialogical relationship. Nor is seeing the other's face an issue. Marcus does ask himself why he is not more generous to others, but he asks from a height above them. I never find him asking what more he can learn from others. The pantheon of those from whom Marcus has learned, and to whom he is grateful, seems to close after book 1 of the *Meditations*.

Christianity, on Starobinski's account, introduces a calculus of exchange into gift giving, thus raising the question of how generous this giving is. The medieval Christian giver—typically the giver of alms to the poor—"makes heaven indebted to him" (90). "Wages are promised in return for his alms. He accumulates a treasure" (90, 94). Theology mandates the vertical economy of the gift—looking upward toward God while reaching toward another human. Starobinski describes the alarm felt by religious censors who saw a scene in Moliére's *Dom Juan* in which the hero gives to a poor man "for the love of humanity." Giving for the love of humanity situates the gift "exclusively in the horizontal dimension" (94). That shift worried the censors, with good reason. An Enlightenment sensibility was evident, bringing another shift in generosity.

Dom Juan gives out of largesse, as a grand gesture of charity, and he gives to his fellow humans without looking up to heaven. The next step is to remove the contingency of charity. Generosity is organized in accordance with principles of equity and efficiency; charity becomes welfare. The Enlightenment, Starobinski writes, "dissociated the question of poverty and the appeal to charity. It made poverty a problem of politics and government" (95). The word *problem* is as significant as the interjection of government between giver and receiver. Neither the ancients nor the early Christians considered giving a problem. Both periods understood giving to be an opportunity, albeit for different ends. The Enlightenment produces "the poor" and "the ill and disabled" as categories of persons who have rights, but these persons become problems; they are no longer faces. The suffering of illness becomes the problem of rising health care costs.

There should be no question of giving up the benefits of the language of rights that the Enlightenment disseminated. The equity of public provision diminishes human suffering by removing many uncertainties that are inherent in private charity (which has its own politics), and by removing the asymmetry that charity signifies. But then people notice that the system—for provision and care no longer happen in discrete personal relationships but now are organized as a system—demoralizes. Being responsible *for* can provide equitable delivery of services, but gone is the generosity that comes from feeling responsible *to*. Hosts become providers, and providers are responsible for only the statutory minimum: what Ignatieff calls "basic needs for food, shelter, clothing, warmth, and medical care" (10). Hosts are responsible to their guests. Providers are responsible to their clients, but they are also responsible to their funders, whether these are taxpayers in a publicly funded system or shareholders in a for-profit system.[4]

"The question," Ignatieff says, observing elderly clients of social welfare in his neighborhood post office, "is whether they get what they need in order to live a human life. . . . What almost never gets asked is whether they might need something more than the means of mere survival" (11). In this book I have tried to ask what "more" is needed. My premise has been that in order to live a *human* life, people need the generosity of their fellow humans. Generosity is what Mr. B needs in the tunnel and after, when he asks what happened; it's what Vanessa Kramer seeks for her aunt after the automatic pain medication machine breaks down; it's what Lori Alvord offers the Begay family when she honors the spirit, not just the formality, of informed consent and lets them have the last word; it's what Linda struggles so hard to offer Mrs. Lambert, and an ideal of generosity is what animates Linda's doubts. Generosity offers something different in each of these stories, but it always begins in dialogue: speaking with someone, not about them; entering a space between I and you, in which we remain other, *alter,* but in which we each offer ourselves to be changed by the other.

When generosity is lacking, that is not because humans have suddenly lost their capacity for it. Modern organizational life, both governmental and corporate, has proliferated a style of being human that was once restricted. This style is the artificial person, and as real as its other values are it transforms generosity from a moral relationship into an administrative problem.

Artificial Persons and Justice

Artificial person is a term revived by philosopher Elizabeth Wolgast to describe how professional and corporate organizations generate dilemmas of moral responsibility.[5] Political philosopher Thomas

Hobbes coined the term in the seventeenth century. Hobbes described artificial persons, or "fictional" persons, as those who "speak and act in the name of others," as governments speak for their citizens or parents speak for their young children. The artificial person also is empowered to "commit and obligate" those others (quoted in Wolgast, 1). Governments, for example, can commit their citizens to paying taxes or going to war. Since Hobbes's time, the number of artificial persons has proliferated. Modern institutions depend on all manner of agents and brokers to speak for and to represent clients, whose consent to be represented is often compelled by necessity. The bureaucrat is an artificial person speaking on behalf of organizational rules and procedures. Bureaucrats are responsible for maintaining these rules and procedures, but not for their effects on clients' lives.

Artificial persons have administrative utility because they act not on their own authority but to implement an authority that resides elsewhere. This usefulness creates the ethical problem that artificial persons no longer feel *personal* responsibility for their actions toward others—they are not supposed to feel such responsibility; others are responsible. Thus as Wolgast writes, artificial personhood "gets in the way of clear assignment of responsibility—and partly for the reason Hobbes gives, namely that the thing done is done in the name of another" (2). The artificial person is no longer responsible as an autonomous individual (what Hobbes calls a "natural person").

Artificial persons can dissociate their actions from their character. Their responsibility is to carry out policies, and to that end they are enjoined not to worry whether they injure their moral souls by acting as they are called to act. Artificial personhood inverts the Stoic framework: people claim their own actions are external; they consider what they do beyond their own control. Nor are artificial persons capable of what Hilde Lindemann Nelson (chapter 1) calls normative self-disclosure. Since their actions are not on their own behalf, they can believe these actions disclose little about themselves as moral beings. How, then, *do* artificial persons express moral awareness and responsibility? At worst, the artificial person is encouraged to claim that responsibility consists in "only following orders," one of the most morally haunting phrases of the last century.[6]

Artificial persons *are* following orders; that's their duty and their honor, and it is also their moral liability. "The important question," Wolgast says, "is whether institutional practice can have priority over moral claims" (3). Wolgast writes mostly about law and the military, but the same dilemmas occur in medical care. *Care* comes to denote a quantity of services expended, not a moral response of one person to another. Care is an allocation, increasingly determined by forms of management. Care derives from state, professional, and private corporate organizations that reach into clinics and hospital rooms through multiple capillaries. Thus for medical workers at the bedside as for soldiers in battle, "Moral ambiguity . . . stems in part from the fact that those receiving the orders are in the circumstances of action while those issuing them stay at a distance" (32). The nurse or physician is face to face with patients, while those determining conditions of treatment remain at a distance. These conditions of treatment include how much time can be spent with a patient, which patients will be referred to specialists and how long they will wait for appointments, and who will pay how much.[7] In these and other matters, the nurse or physician is required to be an artificial person, speaking in the name of the management. Yet professional and personal ethics require responding to this face before you, accepting all the obligation the face commands.

The funniest, and thus cruelest, depiction of the physician as artificial person is presented by Evan Handler in his memoir of his treatment for leukemia. Late in his story Handler has had a bone-marrow transplant. He is in remission from cancer, but his immune system is badly impaired. His central-line catheter (a permanent intravenous line) becomes infected, and he is campaigning, with the support of his nurses, to have it removed before he develops a generalized infection that could be life-threatening, given the impairment to his immune system that resulted from his transplant. Days and nights pass. No surgeon shows up to pull the line. Here is Handler, complaining to his physician, whom he calls Jessica Melman:

"Dr. Melman," I asked. "What is the recommended action for an infected catheter?"

"If the infection can't be cleared, Evan, then the catheter should be removed."

"And if the infection is not cleared and the catheter is not removed, that could be a dangerous situation. Am I right?"

"Theoretically, yes. Of course."

"So, if I have an infected catheter, and it's been three days, and it hasn't been removed, and you can't give me a date and a time when it will be, how is it that I'm receiving adequate care?"

"You are receiving adequate care, Evan," I was told. "Because this is the best care that the hospital can give you."[8]

Dr. Melman presents herself as an artificial person, or in Handler's more colloquial phrase, she is toeing the company line.

David Hilfiker refuses to be an artificial person when he writes how "the limitations" of the clinical environments he works in "require an almost indecent compromise of professional standards."[9] Hilfiker knows what he cannot control, but he also knows his moral soul depends on continuing to speak for himself and taking responsibility for his speech and actions. I cannot evaluate whether Dr. Melman is compromising Handler's safety; she is certainly compromising his care. She is a wary provider, not a host. Her relationship with at least this patient becomes animated by suspicion that is probably mutual, not by generosity and gratitude. Dr. Melman's stance as artificial person puts a wall between herself and her patients, another version of the wall that Ignatieff sees between citizens when layers of government mediation insulate them from one another.

But just as Ignatieff points out the good reasons for that government mediation, so Dr. Melman has good reasons for acting as she does. For us to be able to imagine how to be generous despite the wall of artificial personhood—how to touch each other across and around this wall, since it is probably not going to disappear—we need to understand what the wall serves, and why most of us would not want it to disappear.

The organizational efficiency that results from employees toeing the line is a reason for artificial personhood, but it's not a *good* reason and hardly compensates for the denigration of generosity that is risked. A good reason for the wall of artificial personhood is justice. Justice, as Levinas points out, imposes a limitation on one person's obligation to the face of another. Levinas says, in philosophical language, what we could imagine Dr. Melman wanting to reply to Handler:

If there were only the two of us in the world, you and I, then there would be no question, then. . . . I am responsible to the other in everything. . . . But we are not only two, we are at least three. Now we are a threesome; we are a humanity. The question then arises—the political question: *who* is my neighbor? . . . The other was precisely what I call the "face." For me, he is singular. When the third appears, the other's singularity is placed in question. I must look him in the face as well. One must, then, compare the incomparable.[10]

"There are battered people all over the place!" writes Hilfiker, who wants to be responsible to the face before him but realizes that in some respects, he cannot. "I sometimes wonder what the Good Samaritan would have done if the road to Jericho had been littered with *hundreds* of men beaten by robbers. The demands of justice, at least in this city, are endless." [11] A more prosaic example is Barry Siegler, the internist, not wanting to "open a Pandora's" by asking questions that he knows he should ask his patient. Siegler is being ungenerous, but he may also be practicing justice, because his world too is full of battered people. Siegler must be just toward other patients who are waiting and toward his family, who also wait.

Levinas believes that the implementation of justice requires the intervention of the State (his capitalization). "The State begins as soon as three are present. It is inevitable. Because no one should be neglected, yet it is impossible to establish with the multiplicity of humanity a relation of unique to unique, of face to face." Levinas recognizes that if the State does not impose justice, "charity runs the risk of being wrong." [12] Generosity can go wrong when the chosen one becomes obligated to the first call, or the loudest call, and not necessarily to the call that is most needy. But Ignatieff raises the problem that there is no absolute standard of need: asking who is most needy is like asking who is my neighbor. So justice for Levinas, indispensable as it is, "always has a bad conscience" (194). Acting with a bad conscience may be the fate of professionals who are required by the demands of justice to be less than hosts. This fate is not doom. The Stoics have no problem with the idea of fate. Their question is what character people show in how they encounter their fate.

Dr. Melman's failure of generosity is not her inability to get Handler's catheter pulled; Handler does not know what demands of justice require him to wait. Melman's failure is concealing—certainly to Handler and possibly to herself as well—her own guilty conscience, the inevitable bad conscience of justice. This failure reflects her lack of character, in a Stoic sense. Hilfiker again provides a contrast. What he calls his "brokenness," to which he refers after he asks his rhetorical question about the Good Samaritan, is his guilty conscience in Levinas's sense. This guilty conscience allows Hilfiker to acknowledge the demands of justice—the need of each patient must be balanced against the good of the community of patients—without losing sight of the face of each individual. He breaks between these two demands, but in his acknowledgment of his brokenness, he discovers himself anew and remains generous. Justice does not require taking on a dissociated morality, however much the demands of being an artificial person push humans toward that dissociation. Living with your own brokenness does require faith, whether that's Christian (as for Hilfiker), ancient Chinese (as for Sam Crane), or dialogical.

The Dialogical Stoic, speaking as Marcus Aurelius or as Levinas, upholds an ultimate personal responsibility for remaining generous. Justice can require speaking for others and comparing the incomparable, but the moral soul accepts the guilty conscience, or brokenness, or whatever we call the conflicted stance that implements justice while still seeing the face.

The message of the Dialogical Stoic confronts a new form of artificial personhood that is developing. Hobbes's artificial person gave up personal responsibility in order to accept the responsibility of speaking for some collective that requires leadership. At best (though the worst certainly occurred and maybe more often), that denial was a burden of representing those for whom the artificial person was called to speak: the crown was heavy. Are we now producing artificial persons trained to ignore responsibilities that they offload onto others? Michael Bérubé describes the lesson that children are taught when those who have disabilities, like Bérubé's son Jamie, are removed from classrooms because their presence delays the efficient educational progress of students who are considered developmentally normal. "One thing they'll learn is the implicit lesson I learned as a child: *The 'disabled' are always other people. You don't have to worry about them. Someone else is doing that.*" [13] Those involved in this offloading would probably rationalize it as society's most efficient way to manage people whose needs define them as problems.

The developmentally normal children, now left to progress without distraction, are being taught to become persons who are artificial in their insulation.[14] These modern artificial persons seal themselves off, but not in order to serve an interest beyond themselves, which was the avowed purpose of Hobbes's artificial person. The Stoics seal themselves in an inner citadel in order to serve. They discipline themselves to remain focused on the needs of the human community and to avoid being distracted by what is worst in their fellow humans—qualities they never forget they share, but never give up seeking to overcome. The new artificial personhood serves no comparable ideal, an unanticipated by-product of the state intervention that Levinas describes as necessary. Bérubé would affirm that necessity. The state protects Jamie because it insures justice, which affords Jamie rights. But this justice can easily turn into the belief that "someone else is doing that." Justice can lose its guilty conscience. So Bérubé writes in order to show us Jamie's face, to make readers feel responsible *to* Jamie, not abstractly responsible *for* him. Jamie is the face: weak and vulnerable to changing political whims that become budget allocations. Only a sense of obligation to the face protects Jamie, or Aidan Crane, or the earth, endangered as Terry Tempest Williams shows it to be.

Jamie Bérubé and Aidan Crane are other to the healthy mainstream, just as those of us who live far from nuclear waste want to see those places as other to our backyards. "The question now becomes: what shall we make of this gift of otherness?" asks Bakhtin scholar Michael Holquist, writing on dialogical morality.[15] Justice, when implemented by artificial persons, too readily sees Jamie's otherness only as a problem, not as a gift. Feeling compelled by demands of just distribution to see the person as problem ought to be the guilty conscience of artificial persons. But for them to feel guilty, they would have to see, and the new artificial persons have been trained not to. The issue is not to do away with justice or its need for artificial persons. The issue is how to live with the demands of justice without sacrificing otherness as well as our own moral souls.

OUT OF THE TUNNEL

A dialogical inquiry seeks not to conclude, if conclusion implies synthesis. The Dialogical Stoic fears the pretension of claiming some last word. Bakhtin writes that for those committed to dialogue, "the idea . . . is never cut off from the voice," and since voices remain unfinalized, "there can be no talk here of any sort of synthesis."[16] Synthesis turns unfinalizable dialogue into monologue, because it finalizes others' responses to the world in order to weigh them and add them up. It compares voices that, as Levinas says of the face, are incomparable, in order to order these voices.

If unfinalized generosity resists conclusion, it does require a practice: ways of thinking and acting that, if they become habitual, can make each of us more generous, even in inhospitable institutions. The point of the stories told in this book is not for us to admire their generosity. The stories are hosts, offering us images of our own attainable potential for being generous.

Bakhtin shows how dialogue is a practice of generosity:

> All that matters is the choice, the resolution of the question, "Who am I?" and "With whom am I?" To find one's own voice and to orient it among other voices, to combine it with some and to oppose it to others, to separate one's voice from another voice with which it has inseparably merged—these are the tasks that the heroes solve in the course of the novel. (239)

We might doubt the translation of the singular "question," since Bakhtin asks two questions: "Who am I?" and "With whom am I?" But these two questions are complementary halves of what, in dialogue, is a single question. Dialogue is the complementarity of merging and separating: orienting your voice to others, merging with those other voices, then separating again, and never finalizing this process. Alterity remains in tension with the desire to merge with the other. The heroic task is to live with tension, perpetually seeking balance. This balance solves but never resolves; it is never a finalized solution. What is solved is how to keep the tension within the bounds of dialogue—to keep dialogue open.

Linda is one of Bakhtin's heroes as she tries to solve her relationship with her patient, Mrs. Lambert. Sometimes Linda speaks of Mrs. Lambert as wholly other, assessing her clinical progress. At other moments Linda's judgment seems merged with Mrs. Lambert's. Is Linda describing Mrs. Lambert's doubts or her own when she says "some people may come for their own comfort and not hers"? Is it Mrs. Lambert who pronounces Linda's final judgment: "Sometimes we need to feel we are doing something, but it doesn't help"? Linda struggles not to "overstep" her boundary in either direction. She seeks to avoid straying too far into nonself-sufficiency that becomes merging, and she knows that critical care nursing readily justifies too much distance, leaving the face of the other unseen. The evident ambivalences of Linda's story show that she never resolves this problem. She solves it by carrying on. Her work is the unfinalized process of living with boundary tensions. This process can be chaos, but in this chaos Linda seeks generosity.

Linda is a good nurse because she never loses sight of Mrs. Lambert's face, as Levinas uses that trope: her "exposure to death: the without-defense, the nudity and the misery of the other."[17] Linda's neck spasm is an expression of her responsibility for the face of the other. She does overstep her boundary, but she is acceding to the impossible demand to feel responsible for everything. Linda makes herself hostage to her patient: she is Levinas's "chosen one" who is the "first one called" to care for the other (153). If she goes too far and becomes one of those who want to do something even if it doesn't help, she carries on her struggle to find where that boundary is. That struggle is her moral perfectionism.

Crazy as Levinas's moral perfectionism may be, its practical applicability is evident in Lori Alvord's story, told in chapter 4, of her patient Melanie Begay, whose grandmother will not give consent for surgery. As I wrote the preceding sentence, I almost added: "surgery that she needs." What Melanie needs is for the question of her need to be kept open. To assert that she needs surgery, as if that need naturally trumps all others, would finalize the dialogue as an opposition between the doctor who knows the truth of her patient's need and the family member who has to be brought around to this truth. Alvord never asserts some finalized need as a trump in her dialogue with Mrs. Begay. The Begays' alterity is one side of Alvord's own life and history, and her care for the Begays exemplifies the unity of Bakhtin's dual question of "Who am I?" and "With whom am I?" Alvord's care of Melanie is a process of orienting her voice to the Begays: now it merges with their voices, then it separates so that she can represent Western medicine and all it can offer Melanie. This dialogue continues as Alvord writes about the Begays, giving their alterity a voice on which their face depends.

Alvord represents the Begay family's crazy demand with all the care that Michael Bérubé represents his disabled son, Jamie, knowing that Jamie's future can depend on how he is represented. Alvord intersperses the Begays' story with the history of the Long Walk of 1863, because the present, clinical events cannot be represented without this history, which is a living experience for contemporary Navajo. U.S. troops, led by Colonel Kit Carson, pursued a scorched-earth campaign that starved the Navajo nation into submission. Those who survived were forced to walk three hundred and fifty miles to an internment camp, with massive loss of life along the route and at the camp. Alvord compares this genocide to the Holocaust of European Jewry: "it is the historical event that most illustrates our vulnerability as a race."[18]

Alvord's awareness of this story makes possible her clinical care of the Begays. In this story of vulnerability, she sees the face she shares with the Begay family. She knows Melanie's grandmother, Bernice Begay, probably had a family member on the Long Walk; Mrs. Begay knows who she is, and what she must do, as part of the story of the Long Walk. Alvord recognizes that Mrs. Begay has probably been subject to contemporary government policies that have had similar, if less devastating, effects.

Alvord allows Bernice Begay control over the surgery because the face, and its alterity, demands it. If Alvord were to present a medical argument to save Melanie's life first and sort out people's feelings afterwards, this tactic would reveal only one aspect of Melanie's vulnerability. She is not only sick and in need of surgery. Her face includes her vulnerability as one whose people were forced on the Long March; within this story she will become whoever she is. For Melanie to have a life that is worth living, when surgery saves her life, the alterity of her people must be upheld. Alterity requires giving Melanie's grandmother the last word on whether the white man's medicine can be trusted.

Those who believe the risk of Melanie dying subsumes any risk to Melanie's alterity might meditate on one of Marcus Aurelius's consolations for the ill. Marcus reminds himself that physical diseases can threaten only the duration of his life, and life's duration is beyond anyone's control. He must concern himself with what threatens his *daimōn*, the best part of his character, his moral soul. Lapses of character attack his humanity (ix.2): dishonesty, hypocrisy, and the ease with which a man in his position could act like an artificial person. Marcus expresses the underlying principle that determines how Alvord acts: Physical survival is not the most important value. Or, physical survival is valuable only as a means to continue to express your *daimōn*.

If the moral perfectionism of the Dialogical Stoic is crazy, then Alvord, like Campo, Hilfiker, and Verghese, realizes she has to be no less crazy to be the kind of doctor that her character demands. Part of this craziness is accepting the unfinalized nature of action: acting without certainty of outcome. The stories told in this book are models of acting without reassurance how it will turn out: Alvord waits for Bernice Begay to make up her mind; David Hilfiker runs down a Washington street at night, trying to convince a patient to return to the clinic for treatment; Rafael Campo lets himself acknowledge he loves a patient; Terry Tempest Williams gets arrested in a demonstration; and Vanessa Kramer thinks about declining toxic treatments for cancer. Each does something he or she knows is a bit crazy. Of course there are multiple risks in each of these actions. But these actions are necessary for each to protect her or his *daimōn*. As Levinas writes, to be human "consists in acting without letting yourself be guided by these menacing possibilities. That is what the awakening to the human is."[19]

Allowing ourselves to be guided by menacing possibilities is a symptom of demoralization. I frequently wonder how much the constant barrage of menacing possibilities about health care—menaces usually expressed in financial terms—demoralizes those who work in medical settings, as well as those who enter such settings needing help. When menaced, medical workers withdraw into some form of artificial personhood, a stance that is all too convenient for employers who define efficiency in economic terms and give orders at a distance. Patients respond to their perception of staff by withdrawing into their own suspicion. Menacing possibilities often begin with issues that do require responsive action. These issues become menacing when the range of possible response is artificially limited. Then the menace in the possibility becomes a self-fulfilling prophecy, because the response is already demoralized.[20] The stories in this book show medicine's guests and hosts alike other possibilities are open to us, other stories that provide remoralized imaginations of how we can act.

Refusing to allow ourselves to be guided by menacing possibilities is one demand of moral perfectionism, illustrated in these stories of generosity and elaborated in the Dialogical Stoic's reflections on these stories. The demands of moral perfectionism are as realistic as they are impossible, as Hilary Putnam writes. Putnam argues that "only by keeping an 'impossible' demand in view . . . can one strive for one's 'unattained but attainable self.'"[21] Striving for what is unattainable does not mean reaching that level—the nature of striving is *not* reaching it. Levinas elaborates: "I am not saying that men are saints or that they go toward holiness, I am only saying that the vocation of holiness

is recognized by every human being as a value and that this recognition defines the human." He goes on to say that institutions can never
"assure or even produce holiness." Despite that, or perhaps because of
it, "there have been saints." [22]

David Hilfiker gives the issue a different twist, writing that to practice poverty medicine, "sainthood isn't a prerequisite for the job." [23] He
might argue that we have the wrong idea of sainthood if we imagine
that Fabiola—our presiding figure of saintly generosity—was secure
in her faith and singular in her purpose. Hilfiker may be closer to the
reality of being saintly when he evokes his own brokenness. Perhaps
what is prerequisite for the job is the capacity to tolerate your own internal separations and dilemmas, your losses both real and imagined.
Perhaps brokenness is another name for what I called the diaspora
quality of the physician narratives in chapter 4. Both brokenness and
diaspora denote a condition of irremediable splitting. The moral problem is how to regain, here where we are, what was lost there; and to remember that *there*, either as imaginary homeland or as an imagination
of moral perfection, is unattainable, yet no less real a force in our lives
for being imaginary. Experienced this way, splitting is not alienation;
it's the prerequisite for moral life.

How does each person, each of *us*, act to restore generosity? Responses to this question risk becoming lost in elaborations of institutional complications and menacing possibilities. Marcus is direct, as always: "Everything you're trying to reach—by taking the long way
round—you could have right now, this moment. If you'd only stop
thwarting you own attempts" (Hays, xii.2). [24] Marcus is serious about
our being able to have what we want, right now, but doing that depends
on training. We need a version of the daily practice that Marcus engages in—the practice that includes writing his *Meditations*, which
might have been better titled "Exercises to Stop Thwarting Yourself."
Marcus's practice is to review each day: to recall when he has thwarted
his own attempts and to point out to himself how he can have what he
desires right now. That review is not complete until he has written the
appropriate reminder to himself. Working on the literary style of this
reminder embeds the lesson in how he perceives, thinks, and acts.

Can Marcus's Stoic discipline be adapted to our present needs as
we, guests and hosts alike, try to find what we want in the contemporary medical moment? Generosity is one standard of what we should

want—our unattained but attainable desire. Most of us require training in how to be generous, to ourselves and to others, right now, as well as training to recognize how we thwart our own attempts. Patients and providers are expected to develop all sorts of skills that require training and practice. Why should it require less practice to learn the skills of generosity: how to be good guests and hosts?

Marcus's daily self-questioning revolves around three issues, discussed in chapter 2: perceptions, desire, and action. With respect to his *perceptions,* he trains himself to interrupt the value judgments—condemnation or praise, horror or enticement—that he instinctively associates with what he perceives and to shorten the length of time he is captive to his reactions. Health and illness—both these words themselves, and the situations and bodies they represent—elicit immediate value judgments. We judge our bodies, and our bodies become the measure of our lives, and those judgments impede us. Further value judgments arise when we perceive need—both our own sense of being in need and the need we perceive in others' bodies and lives. These judgments include a sense of what the person in need (who may be me) deserves; is theirs a worthy need? Value judgments lead to attributions of blame and to comparisons: he (or I) did something to create his (or my) own need, she is not as needy as this other person, and so on. Generosity calls on us to interrupt these judgments and to see the need as the suffering it is, an occasion to respond, nothing more. With training, we can perceive suffering, and we can suffer ourselves, without judgment.

With respect to *desire,* Marcus trains himself to suspend his desire for what the world has taught him to consider desirable. He seeks to turn his desire toward what *is:* to desire the present moment just as it is, as part of a cosmos that he cannot understand but can trust. The words *health* and *illness* draw us away from the present into some future that is desired or feared. We need, first, to recognize how often fear is the dark side of desire: much of what we think we desire is to avoid what we fear. Then we need to deal with the immense social machinery—from commercial advertising to nonprofit health promotion to reporting of medical breakthroughs to the imagery and metaphors associated with disease—that seeks to make health synonymous with desire and illness with fear. Marcus cuts this Gordian knot. Desire what is, right now, he tells us. Of course we would rather be healthy, but that will not always happen. So desire above all to be free to live with what is. When you can live with what your own life is, than you can accept the lives of others as they are.

With respect to *action*, Marcus asks himself how well his actions serve the human community of which he is part. He repeatedly reminds himself of being part of this community: no more than one small part, but no less than a fully human part. Does he act as he does to serve others, or as Linda says about those who attend Mrs. Lambert, does he act for his own comfort? Perhaps most important for hosts and guests of medicine is to act without feeling overwhelmed, as Linda is overwhelmed when people need her "all at once." Being ill slows our pace, and caring begins by respecting the pace of those being cared for; instead, institutions expect everyone to speed up. Acting too fast for what the situation requires, we forget that action is a service, to others and to ourselves. We become absorbed in the part that some institution expects us to play and forget our fully human part in a larger community.

Those who are ill and those who work in medicine could well imagine that Marcus is speaking about them when, in one of the passages where he sounds most like Heraclitus, he imagines the world being "like a flood, sweeping all before it." When I have been in deep illness, I have imagined myself caught in that flood, swept along. Part of what floods us are our own expectations, usually for too much. Medical workers and patients are often what Marcus calls, including himself, "little men busy with the affairs of state"; curing and getting cured become things to be busy with. Marcus favors working, but he recognizes that being busy can often prevent the important work from getting done. He tells himself to "get a move on," which means not to expect great things: "be satisfied with even the smallest progress" (ix.29). Medicine, as hyped in mass media and as practiced in complex, expensive institutions, demands return on investment. Marcus recommends seeking satisfaction in the momentary but crucial gesture of personal caring: for yourself, for others, and for the community. I observe that those who have learned to be generous have taught themselves that in order to "get a move on" they need to avoid feeling overwhelmed, and to do that, they need to take pleasure and satisfaction in small progress.

These three, perception, desire, and action, balance each together like legs of a three-legged stool; none comes first and none is the ending. Whether being ill or giving care, act without judgment on your body or the body before you; see it and know it only as what is, as much divinity as dust, part of a cosmos you can trust. Desire what is; don't hook your desire to what you think ought to be—much less to what someone else tells you ought to be—because then you'll end up fearing the failure to achieve that ideal. In health and medicine today, people are trying to sell you ideals; your desire is too often part of being a good customer. Marcus, in his coarse gray cloak, sleeping on his cot, reminds us that we were not put on earth to be customers but to be human. To be human, act with generosity that is content with what it can do—not paralyzed by what is too much for any one person to do, and not forgetting what can be done.

Action, perception, and desire all depend on training. In his *Meditations* that might be better titled "Exercises," Marcus trains himself and shows us how to train ourselves. Did you really think, I can hear him asking us, that the gods have made you fully formed as human? You had to learn to walk and to talk, to respect others and yourself; you had to learn when to seek medical help, and some had to learn how to provide that help. Generosity requires no less training. Get a move on, and be satisfied with that smallest progress by which each of us can move the community toward what our *daimōn* requires.

The Stoic who becomes more dialogical than the ancients could imagine retains Marcus's questions, which are perennial, but can propose five new ones.

First, *dialogue.* "We are two beings," writes Bakhtin, quoted in the first epigraph of this book, "come together." What is this space to which we come, the space between me and an other, and how do I know this space? Perhaps we know the space between by a feeling of having let go of a part of what is conventionally called ego. Bakhtin writes that the dialogical author cedes authority to the character. How do we cede to others some measure of authorship of our lives? And how do we realize, the Dialogical Stoic reminds us, that in allowing other voices to shape our voice, we cede nothing? We only acknowledge what already is and become capable of working with its implications. How do we allow ourselves to be destabilized by others, valuing the otherness that destabilizes what we have so carefully (perhaps too carefully) constructed as stable? What am I to do *here,* in this space between; how does my most important work depend on being here?

Second, *alterity*. We seek what Levinas calls "a kinship for mature persons," which begins in the recognition that however our stories may overlap—and most stories of suffering overlap extensively—our dialogue depends on our differences. Where does my story end and the other's story begin, as a story that is *not* mine? My possibility of responding to the other's suffering, as she or he suffers it, depends on alterity's denial of comparing suffering. Comparison risks symbolic violence; thus Levinas insists that each suffering is unique. Alterity then leads me to one of the most troublesome questions, one that must be asked with the utmost caution: what suffering is rightfully theirs? Not theirs retrospectively, as a judgment on the life this other has lived with its individual choices, or as a result of some collective history this life is embedded in. But theirs prospectively: as the ground of the possibility of that person's future which none of us can yet know. How do I console without limiting the future to which the suffering person has a right? Because alterity measures my distance from my fellow human, it only makes sense side by side with the face, which brings us together.

Third, the *face*. Levinas, in the second epigraph of this book, writes of "the assurance that it is not totally absurd to have suffered." How does one person offer that assurance to another when they meet, "for the last time in the world," as Bakhtin calls such encounters. To prepare for such a meeting, I might ask if I have yet felt the drama of the other's weakness. Do I see the tensions that the other's vulnerabilities create? Do I recognize what the other is having to hold together, to carry on at all, and his or her fear of life coming apart? Then, what part does this other cast me in, in this drama? What part does he or she fear I will play, and what part does he or she hope I might play? What is my obligation—setting aside for the moment all other obligations—to be who this suffering, vulnerable person needs me to be? What response am I called to offer, as if the world depends solely on whether this other person's need was met, and only I could meet it?

Fourth, *justice*. When the needs of third parties require me to compare the needs of persons—to compare what is incomparable—can I acknowledge my guilty conscience? This guilty conscience calls me to render an account for why I have taken the tone of an artificial person: Do I speak in this tone because it makes me a conveniently docile employee, or because it allows me to deny responsibility for my action—

both bad reasons—or because justice demands this tone? How can I be just and not break off dialogue? If I must be an artificial person, can I do so not in self-defense but in a spirit of brokenness? Do I brood when I leave the other because I am needed elsewhere, a leave-taking that the other might experience as abandonment?

These questions *are* questions: not finalized truths but a practice. This practice, unlike most of the history of confessional practices, should be guided by the principle that few of us can be more generous to others than we are to ourselves. *To be generous, first feel grateful.* Each of the storytellers in this book exemplifies this principle. Each discovers that his or her capacity to accept the other depends on, and then enhances, their gratitude for their lives. Generosity and gratitude feed each other. This reciprocity should be joyous, which is the final reflection of the Dialogical Stoic.

Fifth, *joy.* Beyond learning from others, suffering with others, entering a boundary space between me and the other, is there joy in the presence of others? Do I feel pleasure in their presence, and do they seem pleased to be with me? Am I putting up with my fellow humans, as Marcus too often seems to be; do I feel nothing more than responsible for them, which seems a limit for Levinas? What lies beyond Marcus and Levinas is promised by Anatole Broyard's wonderful phrase: that he sought a place where he and his physician could *frolic* together.[25] What have I done, today, to increase the time and space of frolic? We need more stories of frolic; I regret I have offered so few. I hear so few.

All this practice may resolve in a foundational Stoic principle: protect your *daimōn;* and the dialogue corollary: honor the other's *daimōn.* Throughout this chapter I have used the phrase *moral soul.* The soul imagined by the Dialogical Stoic is god-given as a soul-making impulse; acting on this impulse, we create, through our habits, the souls we are. The moral life is enacted in habitual practices that create the generous soul: the soul that knows itself to be in dialogue with other unique souls, that feels obligated to respond to their suffering, that feels joy in their presence. Our *daimōn* is our generosity, our capacity for dialogue, our feeling of being chosen to respond to the suffering of the other, and our joyous gratitude.

In the artworks exhibited in the Louvre's visual history of charity, many of the givers do more than hand over some material gift. These givers place their body among those who receive the gift. Their presence, seeing and touching others, transforms charity into a gift. We who see saintliness made visible in such art then recall that the poor in those pictures had to wait for such a person to bring gifts that would console them for too short a time. The twentieth century did better and worse: offering—when welfare works—some reliable minimum, but often denying the generous presence of a giver and devaluing generosity. Those systems, even where they continue to provide real benefits, are demoralized; a new model is needed.

The generosity that can animate that model is available in the stories of people who have decided that they can be more generous, to themselves and to others. Generosity in this new century begins by giving ourselves to dialogue, to alterity, and to justice. Generosity is giving ourselves to the suffering visible in the face and giving ourselves, no less, to joy. Living in this generosity, we may come to death as Marcus (ii.4) hopes to: grateful to the gods, from the bottom of our hearts.

ACKNOWLEDGMENTS

WRITING this book has given me the privilege to engage people at their very best. My thanks first and foremost to those whose stories I tell. You are Fabiola's true children, keeping generosity alive in our times.

A Killam Resident Fellowship at the University of Calgary, part of the Killam General Endowment Fund, provided me with release from teaching during fall 2002, when most of this book was written. The Killam programs provide major assistance to Canadian academic life, and I am honored to be among their beneficiaries.

My project "Survivorship as Moral Choice," funded by the Social Sciences and Humanities Research Council of Canada, provided additional teaching release and materials. Although this book does not include stories from the interviews that are the core of that research, it does depend on my encounters with people whose commitment to service has been affected by their experience of serious illness.

The Fanny R. Rippel Foundation funded The Hastings Center project "Clinician-Patient Relationships in Cancer Care and Research," which met during the years leading up to this book. Our meetings were a unique opportunity for clinicians, illness survivors, and academics (many of us belonging in multiple categories) to engage in sustained dialogue about medical relationships, especially demands on physicians. Let me thank by name only our organizer, Virginia Ashby Sharpe, though this book continues a dialogue with all my Hastings colleagues.

Other dialogues include those with readers of my manuscript. The first draft was read with sympathetic care by David Morris, Hilde Lindemann Nelson, and Mary Rogers. Their comments were invaluable in my revisions, but their friendship exceeds even what they wrote. Specific chapters were responded to by some of those whose stories are told in these chapters. I hesitate to name them, lest that seem to confer their approval. I could not have written about the people in this book as I have if I did not have the opportunity to know most of them as friends. Another friend, Michael Gardner, introduced me to Bakhtin and gave me the manuscript of his still unpublished reader on dialogical theory. Miles Little, Elliot Mishler, and Alan Radley have each given me specific support and direction.

My thanks to editors and colleagues who have helped me shape my responses to the stories told in this book. Although no previously published writing of mine is included here, I am telling stories that I originally discussed in articles and reviews appearing in *The Hastings Center Report, Health, Qualitative Sociology, Theoretical Medicine and Bioethics, The Christian Century,* and the no-longer-published *Second Opinion.* The core of chapter 1 was originally written for presentation at a conference on narrative-based medicine, convened by Trisha Greenhalgh and Brian Hurwitz and sponsored by British Medical Journal Books. My preparation for a conference on autobiography convened by Paul John Eakin at Indiana University led me to material included in later drafts of chapter 2.

My editor at the University of Chicago Press, Douglas Mitchell, marked his twenty-fifth anniversary with the Press while this book was being written. Our friendship is almost that long, and it's a pleasure to have this book be part of the celebration of Doug's contribution to publishing. My manuscript editor was Sandy Hazel, whose skill is to make her improvements in my text seem like what I was just on the verge of writing myself. But without her, I wouldn't have.

This book echoes conversations with ill people, chaplains and medical professionals, profiteers, politicians, and poets at innumerable conferences over the last dozen years. Some provoked me and others inspired me; each has taught me, and I thank them all. I offer a different sort of thanks to those few friends who shared their current illness experiences with me while I was writing. Every author needs specific imagined readers; thank you for lending your voices and faces.

Finally, thanks to my family: my parents, Jane and Art Frank; my wife, Cathie Foote; and my daughters, Stewart Hamilton Frank and Kate Libbey Foote Frank. Whatever imagination of generosity I am capable of is refracted through my relationships with them.

NOTES

INTRODUCTION

In quoting passages, I decline to insert *sic* to mark gender-biased language of authors, many of whom wrote before it was recognized that *man* is not as inclusive of humanity as other choices of words can be. I leave it to readers to note the publication dates when authors wrote, as well as issues of translation, and decide for themselves whether the gender-biased language is a historical contingency of that period's accepted style or if it represents a flaw in the author's conceptualization of humanity. Where such flaws are evident, the issues are more complex than the insertion of *sic* can resolve.

1. These opening paragraphs draw upon, echo, and consolidate sources from Boethius's *The Consolation of Philosophy* (trans. V. Watts, rev. ed. [London: Penguin, 1999]) to Jacques Derrida's *Adieu to Emmanuel Levinas* (trans. P-A Brault and M. Naas [Stanford, Calif.: Stanford University Press, 1997]). On generosity's forgiving spirit, see David Morris, *Alexander Pope: The Genius of Sense* (Cambridge, Mass.: Harvard University Press, 1984). After completing the first draft of this book, I discovered two crucial discussions of generosity: Rosalyn Diprose, *Corporeal Generosity: On Giving with Nietzsche, Merleau-Ponty, and Levinas* (Albany: State University of New York Press, 2002), and Alan D. Schrift, ed., *The Logic of the Gift: Toward an Ethic of Generosity* (New York and London: Routledge, 1997). Schrift's anthology exemplifies the tension between gift giving as an economy of exchange and the need to imagine generosity outside such an economy.

2. Quoted by Guenter B. Risse, *Mending Bodies, Saving Souls: A History of Hospitals* (New York: Oxford University Press, 1999), 94–95.

3. Abraham Verghese, *The Tennis Partner: A Doctor's Story of Friendship and Loss* (New York: HarperCollins, 1998), 341.

4. For a funny, scathing, and resonant critique of "relentless brightsiding" (49) enforced on breast cancer patients, see Barbara Ehrenreich, "Welcome to Cancerland: A Mammogram Leads to a Cult of Pink Kitsch," *Harper's*, November 2001, 43–53.

5. Or so writes one contemporary translator of a corrupted text that we attribute to the historical but still shadowy figure of Marcus Aurelius. I return to the problem of Marcus's authorship, and our interpretation of his writing, in a later chapter.

6. Northrop Frye, *The Great Code: The Bible and Literature* (Toronto: Academic Press Canada, 1982), 217.

7. The family therapists with whom I have been privileged to work most recently describe their use of reflecting teams in Lorraine M. Wright, Wendy L. Wat-

son, and Janice M. Bell, *Beliefs: The Heart of Healing in Families and Illness* (New York: Basic Books, 1996). Wright, Watson, and Bell focus on the family's beliefs about the issues they face, combining this Stoic emphasis on the ultimate importance of what people believe with a commitment to therapy as dialogue about the value and consequences of holding specific beliefs. Their clinical goal is to enable the family to discover how they want to live and to find the resources to live this way. They do not regard diagnostic labeling of the family's individual and collective pathologies as a useful vocabulary with which to work. For a complementary discussion of a different reflecting-team practice, see Michael White, *Reflections on Narrative Practice: Essays and Interviews* (Adelaide, South Australia: Dulwich Centre Publications, 2000), chap. 4, "Reflecting-Team Work as Definitional Ceremony Revisited."

CHAPTER ONE

1. Richard E. Peschel and Enid Rhodes Peschel, *When a Doctor Hates a Patient and Other Chapters in a Young Physician's Life* (Berkeley and Los Angeles: The University of California Press, 1986), 9–10.

2. Sandra Butler and Barbara Rosenblum, *Cancer in Two Voices* (San Francisco: Spinsters Book Company, 1991), 10.

3. Arthur Kleinman, *The Illness Narratives: Suffering, Healing & the Human Condition* (New York: Basic Books, 1988), 128.

4. Emmanuel Levinas, *Is It Righteous to Be? Interviews with Emmanuel Levinas*, ed. Jill Robbins (Stanford, Calif.: Stanford University Press, 2001), 180.

5. Stephen E. Lammers, "The Marginalization of Religious Voices in Bioethics," in *Religion and Medical Ethics: Looking Back, Looking Forward*, ed. Allen Verhey (Grand Rapids, Mich.: William B. Eerdmans Publishing, 1996), 31. If Lammers seems to reflect a particularly American medical system, and he does, I note the current push in Canada and elsewhere to expand the scope of private, fee-for-service medicine. See Arthur W. Frank, "What's Wrong with Medical Consumerism," in *Consuming Health: The Commodification of Health Care*, ed. Saras Henderson and Alan Petersen (London: Routledge, 2002), 13–30. Note that none of the contributors to *Consuming Health* are American; the commodification issue is hardly specific to American health care.

6. A compelling case for the moral neutrality of medicine is presented by Robert Zussman's ethnography, *Intensive Care: Medical Ethics and the Medical Profession* (Chicago: University of Chicago Press, 1992). Zussman argues that the capacity of intensive care physicians to abstain from moral judgments about their patients is their moral grounding, without which their work would deteriorate into the imposition of personal and cultural biases.

7. John Gardner, *On Moral Fiction* (New York: Basic Books, 1978), 19.

8. "Principlism" has its best-known source in Tom L. Beauchamp and James F. Childress, *Principles of Biomedical Ethics*, 4th ed. (New York: Oxford University Press, 1994). Beauchamp and Childress's four principles are autonomy, beneficence, nonmaleficence, and justice. A cottage industry of publications criticizes and defends principlism. Perhaps most interesting are Childress's own attempts to expand their work to meet different concerns, especially those of critics like Paul Komesaroff and me, who want a greater attention paid to narrative. See James F. Childress, "Narrative(s) Versus Norm(s): A Misplaced Debate in Bioethics," in *Stories and Their Limits: Narrative Approaches to Bioethics*, ed. Hilde Lindemann Nelson (New York: Routledge, 1997), 253–71.

9. Paul A. Komesaroff, "From Bioethics to Microethics: Ethical Debates and Clinical Medicine," in *Troubled Bodies: Clinical Perspectives on Postmodernism, Medical Ethics, and the Body,* ed. Paul A. Komesaroff (Durham, N.C.: Duke University Press, 1995), 65.

10. Paul Komesaroff, personal communication.

11. Robert A. Hahn, *Sickness and Healing: An Anthropological View* (New Haven, Conn.: Yale University Press, 1995), 201).

12. Komesaroff, "From Bioethics to Microethics," 63.

13. Charles L. Bosk, *All God's Mistakes: Genetic Counseling in a Pediatric Hospital* (Chicago: University of Chicago Press, 1992), 171. I quote this story in a different context in *The Wounded Storyteller: Body, Illness, and Ethics* (Chicago: University of Chicago Press, 1995), 147.

14. Mikhail Bakhtin, *Problems of Dostoevsky's Poetics,* ed. and trans. Caryl Emerson (Minneapolis: University of Minnesota Press, 1984), 288.

15. Rachel Naomi Remen, *Kitchen Table Wisdom: Stories That Heal* (New York: Riverhead Books, 1996), 205–6.

16. Hilde Lindemann Nelson, *Damaged Identities, Narrative Repair* (Ithaca, N.Y.: Cornell University Press, 2001), 25.

17. Nelson adapts this phrase from Paul Benson, "Feminist Second Thoughts about Free Agency," *Hypatia* 5, no. 3 (1990): 47–64.

18. See my earlier exploration of this issue, "Interrupted Stories, Interrupted Lives," *Second Opinion: Health, Faith, Ethics* 20, no. 1 (1994): 11–18. See also Gay Becker, *Disrupted Lives: How People Create Meaning in a Chaotic World* (Berkeley and Los Angeles: University of California Press, 1997).

19. Charles Taylor, *Multiculturalism,* ed. Amy Gutmann (Princeton, N.J.: Princeton University Press, 1994), 25.

20. These phrases are Nelson's, *Damaged Identities, Narrative Repair,* 29, 31. On the difficulty of sustaining moral selfhood from a position of postural inferiority, see S. Kay Toombs, "Sufficient Unto the Day: A Life with Multiple Sclerosis," in *Chronic Illness: From Experience to Policy,* ed. S. Kay Toombs, David Barnard, and Ronald A. Carson (Bloomington: University of Indiana Press, 1995).

21. Lance Armstrong, with Sally Jenkins, *It's Not about the Bike: My Journey Back to Life* (New York: Putnam, 2000), 154–55.

22. It's worth noting that at the time Armstrong was treated for cancer, he already had a lucrative career as a cycle racer, but he had not yet won the kind of races that would make him a celebrity outside the niche of his sport.

23. Arthur W. Frank, *At the Will of the Body: Reflections on Illness* (Boston: Houghton Mifflin, 1991). A version of this story is included in the afterword in the 2002 edition.

24. For the complementary view of caring-in-relation by a physician, see Lucy M. Candib, *Medicine and the Family: A Feminist Perspective* (New York: Basic Books, 1995), especially chap. 9.

25. Martin Heidegger, "The Question concerning Technology," in *Basic Writings,* ed. David Krell (New York: Harper & Row, 1977), 297.

26. This argument was clearly stated in 1918 by Max Weber in his lecture "Science as a Vocation." In *From Max Weber,* ed. C. Wright Mills and Hans Gerth (New York: Oxford University Press, 1958), 129–56.

27. On the politics of what counts as "efficiency" in health care, see Janice Gross Stein, *The Cult of Efficiency* (Don Mills, Ontario: House of Anansi Press, 2001).

28. For similar arguments, see Vaclav Havel, *Living in Truth*, ed. Jan Valdislav (London: Faber & Faber, 1986).

CHAPTER TWO

1. Perhaps most notable is Haven Trevino's adaptation of Lao Tzu's *Tao Te Ching*, which he titled *The Tao of Healing* (San Rafael, Calif.: New World Library, 1993). Trevino was living with ALS (see note 4 below) when he adapted each chapter of the Tao to emphasize its relevance to healing.

2. My favorite in the series is Carlos Castaneda, *Journey to Ixtlan: The Lessons of Don Juan* (New York: Pocket Books, 1972).

3. Sam Crane, *Aidan's Way: The Story of a Boy's Life and a Father's Journey* (Naperville, Ill.: Sourcebooks, Inc., 2003), 167.

4. Phillip Simmons, *Learning to Fall: The Blessings of an Imperfect Life* (New York: Bantam Books, 2002). ALS is popularly known as Lou Gehrig's disease, or, more recently, the disease that causes the death of Morrie Schwartz in Mitch Albom, *Tuesdays with Morrie* (New York: Doubleday, 1997). Simmons, throughout his book, generally declines to name his disease, and I recognize the inadequacy of first identifying him with a disease label.

5. Pierre Hadot, *The Inner Citadel: The* Meditations *of Marcus Aurelius*, trans. Michael Chase (Cambridge, Mass.: Harvard University Press, 1998), viii.

6. R. B. Rutherford, "A Note on the Text," in *The* Meditations *of Marcus Aurelius Antoninus*, trans. A. S. L. Farquharson (Oxford: Oxford University Press, 1989), xxvii.

7. For a good example of this style of self-exhortation, see chapter 6, note 24 in the present text.

8. Thus my quotations from Marcus are based on consultation with translators Hays (New York: The Modern Library, 2002), Hadot (note 5 above), Farquharson (note 6 above), Long in both the original edition (London: The Medici Society, 1909; no. 266 of 500 copies, illustrated by W. Russell Flint) and a "corrected" edition (Irwin Edman, ed., *Marcus Aurelius and His Times* [Roslyn, N.Y.: Walter J. Black, Inc., "Classic Club" Edition, 1945]), and Maxwell Staniforth (Middlesex: Penguin Books, 1964). I list these translations in order of my dependence on them. I include the name of the translator, typically Hays, when I have used that version exclusively and it is distinctive from other translations.

Marcus's text was divided by later editors—not by himself—into books and chapters, though the "books" are of chapter length and "chapters" rarely exceed a paragraph. I use a lowercase roman numeral to refer to the book and arabic numerals to refer to the chapter.

9. Simmons, *Learning to Fall*, 13.

10. See Hadot, *Inner Citadel*, 82; also 285.

11. See also Pierre Hadot, *Philosophy as a Way of Life*, ed. Arnold I. Davidson and trans. Michael Chase (Oxford: Blackwell, 1995), and *What Is Ancient Philosophy?*, trans. Michael Chase (Cambridge, Mass.: Harvard University Press, Belknap Press, 2002). The latter became available only as I was finishing the manuscript of this book.

12. Stoic training is compared to its contemporary schools of philosophy by Martha Nussbaum, *The Therapy of Desire: Theory and Practice in Hellenistic Philosophy* (Princeton, N.J.: Princeton University Press, 1994). True to Hays's observation that Marcus Aurelius is not favored among professionals, Nussbaum says nothing about him.

13. Simmons, *Learning to Fall*, 20.

14. Viktor E. Frankl, *Man's Search for Meaning*, rev. and updated ed. (New York: Washington Square, 1984), 86–87.

15. For details of his arrest (which was mostly for the company he kept and involved questions of who had actually written which books) as well as details of the negotiations surrounding his sentencing, see Katrina Clark and Michael Holquist, *Mikhail Bakhtin* (Cambridge, Mass.: Harvard University Press, 1984), 140–45. These pages include my favorite photo of Bakhtin (p. 144), shown as I always imagine him, lying in bed. From 1921 to the end of his life, Bakhtin suffered from osteomyelitis, causing periodic joint inflammations and high fevers. His right leg was amputated in 1938. His bad health probably saved him from a more severe sentence of internal exile and exempted him from military service in World War II.

16. For Bakhtin's life and an overview of his thinking, see Clark and Holquist, *Mikhail Bakhtin*. Most of the extensive literature on Bakhtin develops his influence on literary studies; for critical essays on Bakhtin's contributions to social science, see Michael Mayerfeld Bell and Michael Gardiner, *Bakhtin and the Human Sciences* (London: Sage Publications, 1998). For a theoretical comparison between Bakhtin, Martin Buber, and Emmanuel Levinas, see Michael Gardiner, "Alterity and Ethics: A Dialogical Perspective," *Theory, Culture, & Society* 13(1996): 121–43.

17. Simon Dentith, *Bakhtinian Thought: An Introductory Reader* (London: Routledge, 1995), 41. For the purposes of my present arguments, the validity of Bakhtin's reading of Dostoevsky is not an issue. Bakhtin's "Dostoevsky" could be a kind of character he uses to express his own moral philosophy.

18. Mikhail Bakhtin, *Problems in Dostoevsky's Poetics*, ed. and trans. Caryl Emerson (Minneapolis: University of Minnesota Press, 1984), 63.

19. M. M. Bakhtin, *Speech Genres & Other Late Essays*, trans. Vern W. McGee (Austin: University of Texas Press, 1986), 138. I owe this quotation to Gardiner, "Alterity and Ethics," 137. Cf. Bakhtin's observation on Dostoevsky's characters: "His consciousness of self is constantly perceived against the background of another's consciousness of him—'I for myself' against the background of 'I for another.' Thus the hero's words about himself are structured under the continuous influence of someone else's words about him." *Problems in Dostoevsky's Poetics*, 207.

20. Bakhtin, *Problems of Dostoevsky's Poetics*, 287.

21. Clark and Holquist, *Mikhail Bakhtin*, 78.

22. Bakhtin, *Problems in Dostoevsky's Poetics*, 252. I quote the translation by Clark and Holquist, *Mikhail Bakhtin*, 86. The context of this quotation is a discussion of how Bakhtin translated the religious beliefs of his milieu "into the more widely appropriate discourses of linguistics and social theory" (85), although Bakhtin's continuing belief is a matter of considerable discussion.

23. These biographical details are taken from interviews included in Emmanuel Levinas, *Is It Righteous to Be? Interviews with Emmanuel Levinas*, ed. Jill Robbins (Stanford, Calif.: Stanford University Press, 2001).

24. Emmanuel Levinas, *Difficult Freedom: Essays on Judaism*, trans. Sean Hand (Baltimore: Johns Hopkins University Press, 1990), 291.

25. Levinas, *Is It Righteous to Be?*, 48. Throughout this book I have quoted Levinas's interviews as a matter of literary convenience. His ideas are systematically expressed in his monographs and essays, but brief quotations from these writings make obscure reading. Levinas's syntax often makes for fractured English. He em-

ploys a specialized, philosophical vocabulary, and the sentences are even more difficult when taken out of context. Among Levinas's extensive writings, I find most useful the recent collections of essays, *Entre Nous: Thinking-of-the-Other*, trans. Michael B. Smith and Barbara Harshav (New York: Columbia University Press, 1998), and *Alterity & Transcendence*, trans. Michael B. Smith (New York: Columbia University Press, 1999). Among secondary sources, Jill Robbins, *Altered Reading: Levinas and Literature* (Chicago: University of Chicago Press, 1999) was important to me. My introductions to Levinas were from Zygmunt Bauman, especially *Postmodern Ethics* (Oxford: Blackwell, 1993) and *Life in Fragments: Essays in Postmodern Morality* (Oxford: Blackwell, 1995), and John D. Caputo, *Against Ethics: Contributions to a Poetics of Obligation with Constant Reference to Deconstruction* (Bloomington: Indiana University Press, 1993).

26. A more extended quotation including this phrase is in chapter 3 of the present text.

27. Pascal is a more constant reference than Kafka. Levinas repeatedly quotes Pascal's aphorism that for an individual to claim his "place in the sun" is "the usurpation of the whole each" (Levinas, *Is It Righteous to Be?*, 53; see also 97-99, 205, 225).

28. This description of Buber also represents the American pragmatist tradition and the ethics immanent in sociological symbolic interactionism, e.g., George Herbert Mead, *Mind, Self, and Society* (Chicago: University of Chicago Press, 1934).

29. Bakhtin, *Problems of Dostoevsky's Poetics*, 287.

30. See Levinas, *Is It Righteous to Be?*, 213.

31. On "the original sociality," see ibid., 192.

32. Hilary Putnam, "Levinas and Judaism," in *The Cambridge Companion to Levinas*, ed. Simon Critchley and Robert Bernasconi (Cambridge: Cambridge University Press, 2002), 33-62; the quotation is from 42.

33. Levinas, *Is It Righteous to Be?*, 205.

34. Bakhtin, *Problems of Dostoevsky's Poetics*, 183.

35. Heraclitus, *Fragments: The Collected Wisdom of Heraclitus*, trans. Brooks Haxton (New York: Viking, 2001), 57. Note that this fragment seems to be known only from what Marcus writes, and translations are based on his paraphrase. We never escape the question of whose words these are: in this instance, Heraclitus, Marcus, or some medieval copyist(s), in addition to divergent translators.

CHAPTER THREE

1. Albert Schweitzer, *The Primeval Forest* (Baltimore: Johns Hopkins University Press, 1998), 128. This volume comprises two of Schweitzer's books, *On the Edge of the Primeval Forest* (1921), originally translated by C. T. Campion, and *More from the Primeval Forest* (1931). So far as I can tell, Campion is the translator of the passage quoted, but his translation may have been modified.

2. Albert Schweitzer, *Out of My Life and Thought: An Autobiography*, trans. A. B. Lemke (New York: Holt, Rinehart and Winston, 1933; rev. ed., trans. Antje Bultmann Lemke, with a preface by Rhena Schweitzer Miller and Antje Bultmann Lemke, New York: Henry Holt, 1990), 233; page reference is to the revised edition.

3. Schweitzer, *The Primeval Forest*, 111.

4. Mikhail Bakhtin, *Problems of Dostoevsky's Poetics*, ed. and trans. Caryl Emerson (Minneapolis: University of Minnesota Press, 1984), 120. Bakhtin is ar-

guing that Epictetus and Marcus Aurelius (and later Augustine) were "remarkable masters" of "an active dialogical approach to one's self" that "breaks down the outer shell of the self's image, that shell which exists for other people" and which substitutes self-assessment in the eyes of others for "the purity of self-consciousness." It takes a dialogical thinker to know a Stoic. The question is how far Marcus succeeded in creating a self-consciousness that improved his dealings with others, so long as he retained his "outer shell." He frequently reflects on how much his official position requires from him—passages that physicians might note—and reminds himself not to complain about that. Yet the epigraph to this chapter is taken from a passage that begins with Marcus writing that when his fellow humans are obstacles to him, he is as indifferent to them as to "the sun or wind or a wild beast" (v.20).

5. Schweitzer, *Out of My Life and Thought*, 233.

6. Emmanuel Levinas, *Is It Righteous to Be? Interviews with Emmanuel Levinas*, ed. Jill Robbins (Stanford, Calif.: Stanford University Press, 2001), 165, latter emphases added.

7. Schweitzer, *Out of My Life and Thought*, 195.

8. Hilary Putnam, "Levinas and Judaism," in *The Cambridge Companion to Levinas*, ed. Simon Critchley and Robert Bernasconi (Cambridge: Cambridge University Press, 2002), 36. Putnam borrows the idea of moral perfectionism, and some of his description of it, from Stanley Cavell, *Conditions Handsome and Unhandsome* (Chicago: University of Chicago Press, 1990).

9. Levinas, *Is It Righteous to Be?*, 163.

10. Reynolds Price, *A Whole New Life* (New York: Atheneum, 1994), 182.

11. Price's moral beliefs become more explicit in his later book on illness, *Letter to a Man in the Fire: Does God Exist and Does He Care?* (New York: Scribner, 1999). Although Marcus does not approve of asking why bad things happen, since that implies a prior definition of some things as "bad" (see vi.42, quoted in chapter 1), he would like Price's conclusion on the need to accept suffering as part of a design, and a harmony, beyond human comprehension. For Price: "What if we'd been allowed, in our worship, to grant . . . that a fathering God . . . may be all things, creative and destructive, to his creatures and that each of these things is *good*, whatever our immediate evaluation of it, and good precisely because it is the will of that Father and in some ways fulfills the intent of his ongoing care for all that exists?" (76–77). For Marcus: "Everything is interwoven, and the web is holy; none of its parts are unconnected. They are composed harmoniously, and together they compose the world. One world, made up of all things. One divinity, present in them all" (vii.9).

12. Whether Price's dialogue is within himself depends on the reader's understanding of God. The centerpieces of *A Whole New Life* are two visions that Price has, seeing Jesus in one instance, and hearing what he takes to be the voice of God in another. As argued in chapter 1 of the present text, no firm boundary separates self and other, including God as other.

13. Henry Louis Gates Jr., "'Race' as the Trope of the World," in *Social Theory: The Multicultural & Classic Readings*, ed. Charles Lemert (Boulder, Colo.: Westview Press, 1993), 590–96.

14. See David Rothman, *Strangers at the Bedside: A History of How Law and Bioethics Transformed Medical Decision Making* (New York: Basic Books, 1991). Unfortunately the ritualized requirement to obtain a signature on a release form

does not necessarily presuppose recognizing a face. At least the ideal of informed consent acknowledges that patients can represent themselves; to that extent it transforms their absence into a presence.

15. The literature on disability and representation is vast, but let me honor an early book by a founder of the disability rights movement, Irving Kenneth Zola, *Missing Pieces: A Chronicle of Living with a Disability* (Philadelphia: Temple University Press, 1982). What Zola chronicles is his own developing awareness of the effect of disability on his life, and how he has misrepresented himself to himself in denying that effect. He shows the intertwining of social recognition and self-recognition, and the multiple ways that disability is represented, especially in architecture and physical space. For a more recent exemplary work, see James Charlton, *Nothing about Us without Us: Disability Oppression and Empowerment* (Berkeley and Los Angeles: University of California Press, 1998), a title that speaks directly to the issue of representation.

16. Michael Bérubé, *Life as We Know It: A Father, a Family, and an Exceptional Child* (New York: Pantheon, 1996), xix.

17. The idea of narratability is also operating in Hilde Lindemann Nelson's work, discussed in chapter 1. The capacity of some groups to block other groups' preferred stories about themselves is one aspect of the problem of representation.

18. Anatole Broyard, *Intoxicated by My Illness and Other Writings on Life and Death* (New York: Clarkson Potter, 1992), 45. Broyard's remarks quoted here were initially made at the Pritzker School of Medicine of the University of Chicago in April 1990.

19. For a rich discussion of suffering as a social danger, see Arthur Kleinman, "Experience and Its Moral Modes: Culture, Human Conditions, and Disorder," in *The Tanner Lectures on Human Values, Vol. 20*, ed. Grethe B. Peterson (Salt Lake City: University of Utah Press, 1999), 355–420.

20. Jason Kingsley and Mitchell Levitz, *Count Us In: Growing Up with Down Syndrome* (San Diego: Harcourt Brace and Company, 1994).

21. Kingsley and Levitz, *Count Us In*, 27.

22. Levinas, *Is It Righteous to Be?*, 177. The context is a comment that this fearing for the other is absent in Heidegger's analyses, however brilliant these analyses are. In Heidegger, Levinas asserts, "all emotion, all fear, is finally emotion for oneself, fear for oneself, fear of the dog but anguish *for* oneself." Whether or not that is fair to Heidegger, it's a strong statement of what dialogical morality seeks to move past.

23. Nancy Mairs, *Waist-High in the World: A Life among the Nondisabled* (Boston: Beacon Press, 1966), 60.

24. On the reality of these fantasies, see Timothy Diamond, *Making Gray Gold: Narratives of Nursing Home Care* (Chicago: University of Chicago Press, 1992). Note how for the Stoic, entertaining such fears is a choice, and someone who entertained these fears has failed in the first task of distinguishing what she could control from what she could not. Yet that denial of the body's suffering would be further than Mairs and most people today want to go.

25. For a complementary personal and philosophical reflection on the social dismissal of disabled people, see S. Kay Toombs, "Reflections on Bodily Change: The Lived Experience of Disability," in *Handbook of Phenomenology and Medicine*, ed. S. Kay Toombs (Dordrecht, the Netherlands: Kluwer Academic Publishers, 2001), 247–61.

26. Levinas, *Is It Righteous to Be?*, 193.

27. Nancy Mairs, *Ordinary Time: Cycles in Marriage, Faith, and Renewal* (Boston: Beacon Press, 1993).

28. Mairs, *Waist-High in the World*, 63.

29. Evan Handler, *Time on Fire: My Comedy of Terrors* (New York: Owl Books, 1996), 175; see also 205, and with respect to nurses who invited his participation, 177–78.

30. Tim Brookes, *Catching My Breath: An Asthmatic Explores His Illness* (New York: Times Books, 1994), 283.

31. Paul A. Komesaroff, "From Bioethics to Microethics: Ethical Debates and Clinical Medicine," in *Troubled Bodies: Clinical Perspectives on Postmodernism, Medical Ethics, and the Body*, ed. Paul A. Komesaroff (Durham, N.C.: Duke University Press, 1995), 69.

32. Brookes, *Catching My Breath*, 284.

33. Since Brookes wrote this passage his argument has moved from moral assertion to epidemiological research; see Ichiro Kawachi, Bruce P. Kennedy, and Richard G. Wilkinson, eds., *The Society and Population Health Reader: Income Inequality and Health* (New York: The New Press, 1999). Linkage between the degree of inequality in a society and health at all income levels is controversial, and epidemiologists are concerned to measure health narrowly, in rates of reported disease, not in Brookes's more extensive, even metaphoric terms. Still, the research provides a provocative complement to Brookes's ideas.

34. Terry Tempest Williams, *Refuge: An Unnatural History of Family and Place* (New York: Vintage, 1991), 3.

35. Vanessa Kramer, "Case Story: Cancer Treatment and Ecology—The Long View," *Making the Rounds in Health, Faith, and Ethics* 1, no. 5 (November 6, 1995): 1, 4–5. Kramer's story was part of a series of first-person illness narratives that I edited in the journal *Second Opinion* and its newsletter successor, *Making the Rounds*, both published by The Park Ridge Center, Chicago. I quote Kramer in greater length than other stories because copies of the original article can be hard to locate. *Making the Rounds* has discontinued publication, and The Park Ridge Center has reduced its activities.

36. Cheryl Mattingly, in her ethnographic study of the clinical practice of occupational therapists, calls this process emplotment. Therapists work to gain patients' adherence to a plot within which the objectives and work of therapy make sense. Patients are called upon to act as characters who fit this plot, at least for the duration of therapy. See Mattingly, *Healing Dramas and Clinical Plots: The Narrative Structure of Experience* (Cambridge: Cambridge University Press, 1998).

37. The cancer center might not be the place to develop this narrative, but it is responsible for the transition. In the best of all hospitals, the results of Kramer's aunt's surgery would have been anticipated, and a representative of the palliative care service would have been on hand, starting a new narrative.

38. Marcus might have responded by asking them if they were any busier than he was, and if more lives depended on them. Levinas might ask if they have more loss to confront than he had.

39. Levinas, *Is It Righteous to Be?*, 127. Levinas then switches to philosophical jargon and restates the issue as "the breakthrough of the human putting into question the ontological necessities and the persistence of a being that perseveres in being."

40. Ibid., 132.
41. Kramer, "Case Story," 5.
42. Levinas, *Is It Righteous to Be?*, 127.

CHAPTER FOUR

1. Anatole Broyard, *Intoxicated by My Illness and Other Writings on Life and Death* (New York: Clarkson Potter, 1992), 45.

2. Abraham Verghese, *My Own Country: A Doctor's Story of a Small Town and Its People in the Age of AIDS* (New York: Simon & Schuster, 1994), 65.

3. Alasdair MacIntyre, *After Virtue: A Study in Moral Theory*, 2d ed. (Notre Dame, Ind.: University of Notre Dame Press, 1984), 216.

4. Cf. Hilde Lindemann Nelson's critique of MacIntyre in *Damaged Identities, Narrative Repair* (Ithaca, N.Y.: Cornell University Press, 2001).

5. Nelson coins the term *counterstories* to describe stories that people tell to establish identities outside the oppressive terms of established, culturally traditional narratives. See ibid. The physician stories in this chapter resemble counterstories in some respects, but they complicate the term. They seek to identify what is oppressive about a culturally *privileged* identity that they enjoy, that of physician.

6. Charles Taylor, *Sources of the Self: The Making of Modern Identity* (Cambridge, Mass.: Harvard University Press, 1989), 63.

7. My choice of which physicians I discuss in this chapter thus has parameters, but it also becomes arbitrary, as I realize looking at some physician-authors I omit: not only Oliver Sacks and Rachel Naomi Remen, but also Lucy M. Candib, *Medicine and the Family: A Feminist Perspective* (New York: Basic Books, 1995), Pedro José Greer, Jr., *Waking Up in America: How One Doctor Brings Hope to Those Who Need It Most* (New York: Simon & Schuster, 1999), and John Lantos, *Do We Still Need Doctors?* (New York: Routledge, 1997) and *The Lazarus Case: Life-and-Death Issues in Neonatal Intensive Care* (Baltimore: Johns Hopkins University Press, 2001). Many other medical professionals are living what those discussed in this chapter have a particular ability to write. For one collection of shorter accounts by physicians telling stories of the moral dimensions of their work, see Jeffrey Borkan, Shmuel Reis, Dov Steinmetz, and Jack H. Medalie, eds., *Patients and Doctors: Life-Changing Stories from Primary Care* (Madison: University of Wisconsin Press, 1999). Beyond these books are many physicians who for whatever reason—lack of inclination or sheer fatigue—have not committed their experiences to prose. Finally I acknowledge the limitations inherent in this chapter focusing on physicians, although a nurse receives full attention in chapter 5. Timothy Diamond's study of nursing homes, *Making Gray Gold: Narratives of Nursing Home Care* (Chicago: University of Chicago Press, 1992), makes a compelling case that the most self-conscious moral actors in health care may be the lowest-paid, least-privileged nursing assistants.

8. Rafael Campo, *The Poetry of Healing: A Doctor's Education in Empathy, Identification, and Desire* (New York: Norton, 1997), 37. The paperback edition is titled *The Desire to Heal*.

9. Lori Arviso Alvord with Elizabeth Cohen Van Pelt, *The Scalpel and the Silver Bear: The First Navajo Woman Surgeon Combines Western Medicine and Traditional Healing* (New York: Bantam, 1999), 185.

10. Campo's experience of Cuba is hardly unique; see an essay that influences this chapter throughout: Stuart Hall, "Cultural Identity and Diaspora," in *Social*

Theory: Continuity & Confrontation, ed. Roberta Garner (Boulder, Colo.: West-view Press, 2000), 560–73.

11. David Hilfiker describes what led him to leave Minnesota in his first book, *Healing the Wounds: A Doctor Looks at His Work* (New York: Pantheon, 1985). What was demoralizing in that practice is another story.

12. Probably the single most frightening comment I remember from an under-graduate paper, in more than a quarter century of university teaching, was when a student, without a trace of irony, referred to the "lifestyle" of concentration camp inmates during the Holocaust. The social relations of privilege that have popularized the word *lifestyle* have also made it increasingly difficult for those who have life-styles—at minimum, the capacity to choose how to style their lives—to compre-hend the lives of those for whom survival allows little choice. The Stoic would ar-gue that life always presents choices, but *lifestyle* is the perversion of self-determination into decisions about consumer purchases that are then used to mediate one's evaluation of self and life.

13. David Hilfiker, *Not All of Us Are Saints: A Doctor's Journey with the Poor* (New York: Hill & Wang, 1994), 13.

14. Rafael Campo, *The Other Man Was Me: A Voyage to the New World* (Houston: Arte Publico Press, 1994).

15. Verghese, *My Own Country*, 104.

16. Verghese finds this place, or perhaps the closest to it, in El Paso, Texas. His move there is described in his second book, *The Tennis Partner: A Doctor's Story of Friendship and Loss* (New York: HarperCollins, 1998). He has since moved again, remaining within Texas.

17. Campo, *Poetry of Healing*, 52–53.

18. For an extensive discussion of the issue of intentional self-infection with HIV, see Walt Odets, *In the Shadow of the Epidemic: Being HIV Positive in the Age of AIDS* (Durham, N.C.: Duke University Press, 1995).

19. Hilfiker, *Not All of Us Are Saints*, 23.

20. See the discussion of Bakhtin in chapter 2.

21. Hilfiker develops this theme in his recent thinking, which depends heav-ily on the writings of philosopher René Girard, especially *The Scapegoat*, trans. Yvonne Freccero (Baltimore: Johns Hopkins University Press, 1986) and *Things Hidden since the Foundation of the World*, trans. Stephen Bann and Michael Met-teer (Stanford, Calif.: Stanford University Press, 1987). Hilfiker's unpublished notes on Girard have informed my interpretive emphasis.

22. Hilfiker, *Not All of Us Are Saints*, 123.

23. Quoted in full above; see chapter 3, note 2.

24. Alvord, *The Scalpel and the Silver Bear*, 12.

25. Cf. 178, when Alvord experiences a complicated delivery of her first child: *"I will have to remember this degree of misery when I am treating sick patients,* I thought. *I will have to remember the way senses are altered."* The latter observa-tion is especially acute and too seldom noted. Medicine, especially biomedical eth-ics, tends to separate the patient's mind, with which business must be conducted, from his or her body. I think especially of women who have had major surgery in the C-section deliveries of their babies, and then are immediately required to make complex decisions regarding the treatment of their impaired infants in neonatal in-tensive care. Bioethics has little recognition for "the way senses are altered" by ill-ness and medical intervention.

26. Mikhail Bakhtin, *Problems of Dostoevsky's Poetics*, ed. and trans. Caryl Emerson (Minneapolis: University of Minnesota Press, 1984), 251.

27. Campo, *Poetry of Healing*, 29.

28. Bakhtin, *Problems of Dostoevsky's Poetics*, 202.

29. M. M. Bakhtin, *Art and Answerability: Early Philosophical Essays*, trans. Vadim Liapunov and ed. Michael Holquist and Vadim Liapunov (Austin: University of Texas Press, 1990), 102.

30. Hall, "Cultural Identity and Diaspora," 571.

31. Hilfiker, *Not All of Us Are Saints*, 22.

CHAPTER FIVE

1. Mikhail Bakhtin, *Problems of Dostoevsky's Poetics*, ed. and trans. Caryl Emerson (Minneapolis: University of Minnesota Press, 1984), 88; Bakhtin is referring to Raskolnikov, the hero of *Crime and Punishment*. The quoted section at the end is from *The Brothers Karamazov;* Alyosha describes Ivan as someone who doesn't "need millions" but just needs "to get a thought straight" (Bakhtin, 87).

2. Linda's story is taken from David Barnard, Anna Towers, Patricia Boston, and Yanna Lambrinidou, *Crossing Over: Narratives of Palliative Care* (New York: Oxford University Press, 2000), chap. 10, narrated by Anna Towers.

3. Bakhtin, *Problems of Dostoevsky's Poetics*, 21.

4. The term *palliative care* overlaps with *hospice care*. *Palliative care* is sometimes used more specifically to refer to the palliation of physical distress, primarily but not exclusively pain, caused by the terminal disease; and *hospice* sometimes refers specifically to the organization of services either in the dying person's home or in a dedicated facility. This chapter uses *palliative care* as the generic term, because that usage follows *Crossing Over*. As a generic term, *palliative care* refers to the withdrawal of invasive medical attempts to cure, provision of the optimal balance of pain control and lucidity, care for the family as well as the patient (and attention to family relationships), and care for the emotional and spiritual needs of the dying person, in addition to providing comforts that are not part of usual hospital care. My discussion of palliative care draws on my own observational experiences during time I spent in the community hospice in Dunedin, New Zealand, and on both writings and personal acquaintance of the following: Ira Byock, *Dying Well: The Prospect for Growth at the End of Life* (New York: Riverhead Books, 1997), Maggie Callanan and Patricia Kelly, *Final Gifts: Understanding the Special Awareness, Needs, and Communications of the Dying* (New York: Bantam Books, 1993), and Michael Kearney, *Mortally Wounded: Stories of Soul Pain, Death, and Healing* (New York: Touchstone, 1996) and *A Place of Healing: Working with Suffering in Living and Dying* (Oxford: Oxford University Press, 2000). An especially useful history is Neil Small and Penny Rhodes, *Too Ill to Talk? User Involvement and Palliative Care* (London: Routledge, 2000).

5. Bakhtin, *Problems of Dostoevsky's Poetics*, 16.

6. Tzvetan Todorov, *Mikhail Bakhtin: The Dialogical Principle*, trans. Wlad Godzich (Minneapolis: University of Minnesota Press, 1984), 107–8.

7. Many social scientific observers of medicine have noted this tendency; see, for example, Robert Zussman, one of the most sympathetic observers: "The very complexity of caring for acutely ill patients takes on something of the character of a game. And in much the same spirit as they would approach a crossword or jigsaw puzzle, many of the interns and residents come to treat patient care much as they

would approach a game." *Intensive Care: Medical Ethics and the Medical Profession* (Chicago: University of Chicago Press, 1992), 58.

8. Barnard and others, *Crossing Over*, 182.

9. Emmanuel Levinas, *Is It Righteous to Be? Interviews with Emmanuel Levinas*, ed. Jill Robbins (Stanford, Calif.: Stanford University Press, 2001), 49.

10. For a detailed exposition of alterity in clinical practice, see Paul Komesaroff, "The Many Faces of the Clinic: A Levinasian View," in *Handbook of Phenomenology and Medicine*, ed. S. Kay Toombs (Dordrecht, The Netherlands: Kluwer Academic Publishers, 2001), 317–30.

11. Bakhtin, *Problems of Dostoevsky's Poetics*, 176.

12. Jean Starobinski, *Largesse*, trans. Jane Marie Todd (Chicago: University of Chicago Press, 1997), 157.

13. M. M. Bakhtin, *Speech Genres and Other Late Essays*, trans. Vern W. McGee (Austin: University of Texas Press, 1986), 138.

14. Starobinski, *Largesse*, 157.

15. Bakhtin is quoting B. M. Engelhardt. *Problems of Dostoevsky's Poetics*, 6.

16. Levinas, *Is It Righteous to Be?*, 166.

CHAPTER SIX

1. Michael Ignatieff, *The Needs of Strangers* (New York: Penguin Books, 1984), 10.

2. For a statement that is classic in its mature ambivalence between appreciating what social welfare policies continue to achieve, and still recognizing the problems associated with welfare as policy, see Michel Foucault's interview, "The Risks of Security," in *Power: The Essential Works of Foucault, 1954–1984*, ed. James D. Faubion (New York: The New Press, 2000), 365–81. Foucault, in that interview, deals with different sorts of risks than I present in this book.

3. Jean Starobinski, *Largesse*, trans. Jane Marie Todd (Chicago: University of Chicago Press, 1997), 90.

4. The concept of shareholder is illustrated in an oral history written by physician Fitzhugh Mullan, based on interviews with Sam Ho, physician and "corporate medical director of a company that employs tens of thousands of physicians under contract to provide health care to 4.5 million people in eleven states and Guam" (138). Ho responds to criticism that corporate salaries in health maintenance organizations are too high: "If an executive brings shareholder value to a corporation measured in billions of dollars, then executive compensation in the few million dollar range is competitive with other industries, and a relative pittance, compared with what the executive has earned for the shareholder. It's a concept of compensating leadership based on added market value." Fitzhugh Mullan, *Big Doctoring in America: Profiles in Primary Care* (Berkeley and Los Angeles: University of California Press, 2002), 146. The contested issue is whether this increased shareholder value—increase in the price of the stock—eventually returns to patients as lower premiums and increased access to more services, or whether patients pay higher premiums and endure restricted services so that executives can increase shareholder value.

5. Elizabeth Wolgast, *Ethics of an Artificial Person: Lost Responsibility in Professions and Organizations* (Stanford, Calif.: Stanford University Press, 1992).

6. For Wolgast's brief discussion of this defense presented by Nazi war criminals at the Nuremberg trials, see ibid., 31, 39.

7. One of the most contentious issues among these conditions of treatment that are beyond medical workers' control is access to patients' medical records. Legislation to protect privacy of medical information will be perpetually catching up with new information technologies that make computerized files difficult to protect; changes in medical knowledge that give information unexpected relevance to different groups; and changes in medical financing, in which people will be required to consent to administrative access to their files as a condition of qualifying for some benefit. Information will continue to be exchanged in a clinical milieu of suspicion that has nothing to do with the trust between the persons for whom that information counts here and now.

8. Evan Handler, *Time On Fire: My Comedy of Terrors* (New York: Henry Holt and Company, 1996), 226.

9. David Hilfiker, *Not All of Us Are Saints: A Doctor's Journey with the Poor* (New York: Hill & Wang, 1994), 213.

10. Emmanuel Levinas, *Is It Righteous to Be? Interviews with Emmanuel Levinas*, ed. Jill Robbins (Stanford, Calif.: Stanford University Press, 2001), 133; see also 115, 165, 214.

11. Hilfiker, *Not All of Us Are Saints*, 169.

12. Levinas, *Is It Righteous to Be?*, 194.

13. Michael Bérubé, *Life As We Know It: A Father, a Family, and an Exceptional Child* (New York: Pantheon, 1996), 204.

14. The distraction caused by children with special needs should not be minimized, and Bérubé, like Sam Crane, would argue that funding must be provided for aides for these children. Generosity is not cheap, but we often fail to consider the moral costs of exclusion.

15. Michael Holquist, introduction to Bakhtin, *Art and Answerability: Early Philosophical Essays*, trans. Vadim Liapunov (Austin: University of Texas Press, 1990), xix.

16. Mikhail Bakhtin, *Problems of Dostoevsky's Poetics*, ed. and trans. Caryl Emerson (Minneapolis: University of Minnesota Press, 1984), 279.

17. Levinas, *Is It Righteous to Be?*, 48. Full quotation in chapter 2, of the present text.

18. Lori Arviso Alvord with Elizabeth Cohen Van Pelt, *The Scalpel and the Silver Bear: The First Navajo Woman Surgeon Combines Western Medicine and Traditional Healing* (New York: Bantam, 1999), 142.

19. Levinas, *Is It Righteous to Be?*, 175.

20. Not only governments and corporations delimit the future of health care as choices between menacing possibilities. I have found it difficult to be as enthusiastic as I once was in support of health charities and illness advocacy groups, because they often adopt the language of threat as how they represent illness and care to the public. To adapt a phrase, I doubt if the tools of demoralization can be used to rebuild a demoralized house. See Audre Lorde, *Sister Outsider* (Freedom, Calif.: The Crossing Press, 1984), 112.

21. Hilary Putnam, "Levinas and Judaism," in *The Cambridge Companion to Levinas*, ed. Simon Critchley and Robert Bernasconi (Cambridge: Cambridge University Press, 2002), 36.

22. Levinas, *Is It Righteous to Be?*, 220.

23. Hilfiker, *Not All of Us Are Saints*, 188.

24. Marcus also writes: "Snotty little men! Man, what must you do? Do what Nature asks you to do in this very moment. Direct your will in this direction, if it

is granted you to do so, and don't look around to see whether anyone will know about it. Don't wait for Plato's Republic! Rather, be content if one tiny thing makes some progress, and reflect on the fact that what results from this tiny thing is no tiny thing at all!" (Hadot, ix, 29) For discussion see Pierre Hadot, *The Inner Citadel: The* Meditations *of Marcus Aurelius,* trans. Michael Chase (Cambridge, Mass.: Harvard University Press, 1998), 303 ff.

25. Anatole Broyard, *Intoxicated by My Illness and Other Writings on Life and Death* (New York: Clarkson Potter, 1992), 45 (quoted in full in chapter 4).

INDEX

AIDS, 79–80, 88–89, 90–92, 102;
physicians' fears of infection from,
87–88, 90–91
alterity: defined, 115; as gift, 132;
training for, 141. *See also under*
Levinas, Emmanuel
Alvord, Lori Arviso, 79, 84, 95–98,
105, 157n25; and Begay family,
96–99, 100, 115–16, 134–36
Armstrong, Lance, 26, 55
artificial person, 126–32; justice as
reason for, 129

Bakhtin, Mikhail, 43–47, 50, 57, 68,
99, 102, 103, 117, 140; biography
of, 43–44, 151n15; on death, 20,
47, 111; on dialogue, 20, 44, 52, 94,
101, 109, 133; Dostoevsky depicted
by, 44, 100, 151n17; on humiliation, 22; and monological voice, 45,
103, 109, 112, 114, 118; and nonself-sufficiency, 46–47, 50, 112–
14, 133, 151n19; and polyphony,
100, 110; on self, 45–46, 119; on
Stoicism, 152n4; on suffering, 104;
on unfinalizability, 46 (defined),
100, 101, 113, 132, 134, 135–36
Begay, Melanie and Bernice. *See under*
Alvord, Lori Arviso
Benedictines, 9; and Rule of St. Benedict, 3
Bérubé, Michael, 61–64, 72, 100,
131–32
Bérubé, Jamie, 64
Bosk, Charles, 21–22
boundaries. *See under* dialogue
Brookes, Tim, 68–69, 76

Broyard, Anatole, 63–64, 78–79, 83,
88, 103, 142
Buber, Martin, 50

Campo, Rafael, 79, 83–84, 89–92, 93,
97, 99, 101–3, 114–15, 136; *The
Other Man Was Me*, 87
care: 4, 27, 128; doubts about, 118–
20; polyphonic, 111; types of,
112–13
Carson, Colonel Kit, 134
Castaneda, Carlos, 30–31
Catholic Workers, 65–66
Clark, Katrina, 46
consolation, 2, 35, 40
Crane, Aidan. *See* Crane, Sam
Crane, Sam, 30, 39–40, 43, 52, 132
Crossing Over (Towers), 108

daimōn, 40, 42, 135, 136, 142
death, 20, 38, 40–41, 74, 76, 102, 111,
114, 122. *See also under* Bakhtin,
Mikhail
Dentith, Simon, 44
Dialogical Stoic, 8, 9, 31–33, 52–54,
110, 131, 132, 135, 136, 140
dialogue, 20, 24–25, 44–47, 77, 98,
109, 113, 118–19; alterity in, 116;
boundaries in, 46, 112–14, 117,
120, 133; incapacity for, 113; necessity of, 53; physical (nonlinguis-
tic) expression of, 32–33, 52, 100;
polyphony and, 100, 110; quarrel
as, 100; training for, 140. *See also*
Bakhtin, Mikhail
Diamond, Timothy, 156n7
Diaspora, 104–5

disability rights, 38, 62–68, 131–32, 154n15
Dom Juan (Moliére), 125
Dostoevsky, Fyodor, 44–45, 49, 61. See also under Bakhtin, Mikhail
Down syndrome, 61, 64

emotional pain. See under palliative care
empathy, 112–13
Epictetus, 37
ethics: versus moral, 19. See also under medicine

Fabiola, 3, 6, 25, 57, 137
face: training for, 141. See also under Levinas, Emmanuel
Farquharson, A. S. L., 34
Frankl, Viktor, 41–42
Frye, Northrop, 7

Gardner, John, 16
Gates, Henry Louis Jr., 60–61
generosity: as charity, 125; Christian, 125; denigration of, 126; as dialogue, 133, 142; doubts associated with, 2, 106, 119–20; financial costs of, 160n14; gratitude compared to, 1, 142; historical periods of, 124–26; improper occasions for, 130; literary form of, 60; versus rights, 123–25; Stoic, 124; training for, 137–143; welcome as, 1–2; welfare as, 123–126. See also medicine, hospitality of; nursing, generosity of

Hadot, Pierre, 33–34, 37–38, 40; on universal Stoicism, 41–42, 53
Hahn, Robert, 21. See also Siegler, Barry
Hall, Stuart, 104–5
Hancock, John, 60
Handler, Evan, 67–68, 128–30
Havel, Vaclav, 28–29, 42
Hays, Gregory, 34–36
healing, 27–29, 77
health care system, 29
health ecology, 68–77

Heidegger, Martin, 28. See also under Levinas, Emmanuel
Heraclitus, 40, 54, 74, 139
Hilfiker, David, 79, 84–87, 92–95, 97, 102, 105, 129, 130, 136, 137; on brokenness, 95–96, 137; on identification with the poor, 92–93, 98; on poverty medicine, 85–86. See also physicians, identification of, with the ill
HIV. See AIDS
Hobbes, Thomas, 126–27. See also artificial person
Holocaust, 41, 51, 58, 135, 157n12. See also Levinas, Emmanuel
Holquist, Michael, 46, 132
hospice care. See palliative care
hypergoods. See under Taylor, Charles

identification with the ill. See under physicians
identification with the poor. See under Hilfiker, David
Ignatieff, Michael, 123–24, 129, 130
illness, 4–5, 32, 55–77; and metaphor of tunnel, 14; as "relentless brightsiding" (Ehrenreich), 147n4; representations of, 60–64. See also physicians, identification of, with the ill

Jerome, 3. See also Fabiola
Job, 2
justice, 51, 129; training for, 141. See also under Levinas, Emmanuel

Kingsley, Jason, 64
Kleinman, Arthur, 15
Komesaroff, Paul, 18, 69, 159n10
Kramer, Vanessa, 69, 71–77, 97, 136

Lambert, Miriam. See Linda
Lammers, Stephen, 15–17
Levinas, Emmanuel, 15, 48–52, 57, 58, 64, 66, 67, 69, 76–77, 94, 122, 136–37, 142; and alterity, 114–18, 134–35; biography of, 48; and face, 48–49, 61, 66, 77, 93–94, 116, 129, 134; on Heidegger, 154n22; on justice, 51, 129–30; "menacing

possibilities" of, 136, 160n20; and
symbolic violence, 115. *See also* al-
terity; dialogue
Levitz, Mitchell, 64
lifestyle, idea of, 157n12
Linda (pseud.), 106–22, 133, 139
Long, George, 34
Long Walk of 1863, 134–35

MacIntyre, Alasdair, 81, 104
Mairs, Nancy, 64–68
Marcus Aurelius, 6, 33–43, 54, 57, 74,
94, 135, 142, 160n24; action, training of, 139; consolation of, 35, 40;
on death, 40–41; desire, training
of, 138–39; generosity of, 125;
gratitude of, 143; *Meditations*,
33–34, 43, 137, 150n8; perception
theory of, 37–40; on training,
40–41, 137–40. *See also daimōn*
Mattingly, Cheryl, 13n36
medical information, problems of,
160n7
medicine: chart talk in, 118; demoralization caused by, 15, 20, 75,
83–84, 85, 90, 95–96; demoralization of patients by, 9, 15, 22, 96,
157n25; ethics of, 18, 98, 148n8,
153n14; efficiency in, 28; fundamental, 1; hospitality of, 1, 3, 6;
hospitals and, 3, 27, 72–73; managed care in, 3, 79, 124, 128, 159n4;
moral power of, 16–17, 80–81, 86;
pain control in, 72–73, 107; reform
of, 29; remoralization of, 25,
28–29; symbolic violence risk in,
116–17; and technology, 28; usage
of word, 10. *See also* nursing; physicians
Moliére, Jean Baptiste Poquelin: *Dom
Juan*, 125
monologue: defined, 45. *See also*
Bakhtin, Mikhail, and monological
voice
moral fiction, 16
moral moments, 19
moral nonfiction, 77
moral perfectionism, 57–58, 134, 135,
136

narratability of stories, 62
narration styles, 109
Nelson, Hilde Lindemann: and counterstories, 156n5; and normative
self-disclosure, 23, 29, 127; and oppressive identity, 23, 28–29
nursing, 110, 133; chaos in, 118, 122;
generosity of, 117; and the good
nurse, 121–22, 134. *See also*
medicine

otherness. *See* alterity; Levinas, Emmanuel

palliative care, 111, 118–20; defined,
158n4; doubts within, 118–20;
emotional pain and, 117–18; preferred story of, 107
Percy, William Alexander, 35
Peschel, Enid Rhodes, 12
Peschel, Richard, 12, 17, 18–21, 23, 25,
39
physicians: demoralization of, 5, 15,
22, 136; education and training of,
20, 75, 83–84, 90, 95–96; generosity of, 16–17, 26, 67, 80, 88–89,
92, 94–104, 115–16, 134–36;
identification of, with the ill, 99,
100, 103; loneliness among, 4
polyphony. *See under* Bakhtin,
Mikhail
Price, Reynolds, 59–60, 153nn11–12
Putnam, Hilary, 51–52, 57, 136

reflecting team, 7–8, 31
*Refuge: An Unnatural History of Fam-
ily and Place* (Williams), 70–71
Remen, Rachel, 22–23
Risse, Guenther, 3
Rosenblum, Barbara, 14–15, 36, 38,
48–49, 53
Rutherford, R. B., 33–34

Schweitzer, Albert, 55–58, 94; on fel-
lowship with pain sufferers, 55–56,
69, 91
Siegler, Barry (pseud.), 21, 120, 130
Simmons, Philip, 33, 35, 37–38
Smith, Bill (pseud.), 21–22

Starobinski, Jean, 119, 124–26
Stoicism, 154n24; and fate, ideas of,
130; generosity of, 124, 131; inver-
sion of, by artificial persons, 127.
See also Marcus Aurelius; Hadot,
Pierre
stories: creating one's own, 81–82;
moral imagination in, 105; resisting, 83; resonance of, 7; as teaching
how to live, 7; thinking *with*, 6–7
suffering. *See under* Bakhtin, Mikhail

Taylor, Charles, 24; and hypergoods,
82, 87, 97
Todorov, Tzvetan, 112
Towers, Anna, 107, 109; *Crossing
Over*, 108
training, 36, 54, 138, 140. *See also under* generosity

"Tunnel, The" (Peschel), 12, 53, 63.
See also Peschel, Richard

Verghese, Abraham, 4, 79–80, 84–85,
87–89, 105

Wheatley, Phillis, 60–61, 64
When a Doctor Hates a Patient
(Peschel and Peschel), 12
Williams, Terry Tempest, 69–71, 76,
132, 136; *Refuge: An Unnatural
History of Family and Place*, 70
Wolgast, Elizabeth. *See* artificial
person
Wright, Lorraine M., 147n7

Zussman, Robert, 148n6, 158n7